Hormone Powered

Hormone Powered

The Ultimate Guide to Radiant Health in Your 20s, 30s, 40s, and Beyond

Corina Dunlap, ND, MS

JOSSEY-BASS™
A Wiley Brand

Published by John Wiley & Sons, Inc., Hoboken, New Jersey.

For general information on our other products and services or for technical support, please contact our Customer Care Department within the United States at (800) 762-2974, outside the United States at (317) 572-3993 or fax (317) 572-4002.

Wiley also publishes its books in a variety of electronic formats. Some content that appears in print may not be available in electronic formats. For more information about Wiley products, visit our web site at www.wiley.com.

Library of Congress Cataloging-in-Publication Data is Available:

ISBN 9781394380909 (Cloth)
ISBN 9781394380923 (ePDF)
ISBN 9781394380916 (ePub)

Cover Design and Image: Meghan Lambert
Author Photo: Monica Justesen

SKY10162285_071326

For my daughters, Madeleine and Emilia.

May you always be in awe of your extraordinary bodies and honor the full potential they hold.

May you surround yourself with people who truly care for your well-being, receive guidance from those who can support you, and trust your inner compass above all else.

May you always come to know your most radiant selves and let that light guide you, and others, home.

I love you.

Disclaimer

The purpose of this book is to educate you about your hormones, the functions they perform in your body, what happens when hormone levels get too high or too low, and how to restore hormonal balance with a holistic plan, which may or may not include medication and/or hormone replacement therapy, depending on your unique situation.

The information in this book is intended for educational purposes and not as medical advice. Although I am a licensed naturopathic doctor (ND) and a medical researcher, reading a book is not the same as meeting with a healthcare professional one-on-one and does not constitute me being your doctor.

Please use this book to become informed and empowered about your own body and to guide your choices, alongside recommendations from your healthcare team.

Contents

Introduction: You're Not Broken. You're in the Gap

"What brings you in today?" I asked, greeting my new patient.

She looked sullen and depleted. Dark circles under her eyes. The energy emanating from her body was that of someone defeated and hopeless.

That's when I glanced down and noticed the scars on her arms and wrists. Painful memories, visible in plain sight.

Claudia, a woman in her late 30s, fidgeted in her seat, shoulders caved in, uncomfortable in her own skin. I could almost read her mind: *"I've seen so many specialists before, but I still don't feel okay. Will this be any different?"*

By the time she arrived at my practice, she had spent years on high-dose antidepressants and anxiolytics. Sadly, things had gotten so bad that she had moments of trying to end her life. Feeling like she and her doctors had tried everything, she came to me, a naturopathic doctor with a focus on women's hormones, as a last resort.

Claudia told me what she had been experiencing: chronic infections, depression, anxiety, other diagnoses, including ADHD, difficulty focusing, brain fog, fatigue, and the list went on. She was in rough shape. And I knew that, simply based on her age, significant hormonal changes were ahead; her life wasn't going to get easier.

I began gently asking questions about her health history. Through our conversation, I learned that she hadn't had a regular period in years. Birth control was the only solution ever offered, something she'd try in short bursts, desperate to feel better, only to stop again when it made her mood and everything worse.

Her gynecologist said the pill would "regulate her period" but never mentioned some of the possible side effects, including mood changes. Her psychiatrist wrote various prescriptions, too, but never spoke to Claudia about how hormonal and mental health are deeply interwoven.

In all her years of suffering, none of the providers on her team ever said, "Let's run some tests to check your hormone levels." It never even came up. Not once.

Hearing Claudia's story, I suspected what might be going on. A panel of lab tests confirmed it: *premature ovarian insufficiency*. It's something I see in my practice more and more often. An early shift into perimenopause, cycling in and out of subsequent estrogen and progesterone deficiency, nutrient deficiencies, cortisol dysregulation, and a cascade of hormonal chaos, affecting her skin, her gut, her sleep, her libido, and layers upon layers of impact to her relationships, career, family, and will to live. Claudia's distress didn't happen all at once. It was a gradual decline. A missed diagnosis, more medications that didn't make her feel better, more side effects, and more distance from her true nature, her true personality, her true light.

One thing that I know to be true, deep in my bones, is that our life and health are made up of a collection of moments. Our reality is a culmination of these moments. Like a snowball rolling down a hill, gathering speed, getting bigger and bigger, growing in momentum, each moment builds on the next.

Depending on the choices we make and the care we receive, it can be a positive snowball, or in Claudia's case, a negative one. Her snowball had been rolling in a negative direction for so long that it was turning into a deadly avalanche. Her body was screaming for help.

Yet, no one looked at the whole picture. No one connected the dots. No one offered her hormone testing and truly preventative holistic wellness strategies. No one truly saw her or recognized what was underneath it all: *hormonal dysregulation* that had been escalating for years.

Why Are So Many Women Unwell?

You might not be in a state of extreme distress like Claudia was. Maybe you just feel tired, irritable, foggy, bloated, a bit anxious, somewhat depressed, or "off" in some other way. Not in agony, but not "great" either. Maybe you've been working with a traditional medical doctor, psychiatrist, or both, but aren't noticing much improvement.

Why are millions of women stuck in this state of feeling unwell? Why, despite so many modern advancements in medicine, do so many of us still feel "not great," "mediocre," or even "bad"? And why do so many health conditions, especially those that stem from hormonal causes, get overlooked, dismissed, misdiagnosed, or mistreated?

There are four culprits that, when combined, create a deficiency in the way we care for women in our society. These four contributing factors are a gap in research, a gap in knowledge, a gap in care, and a resulting gap in confidence. To help millions of women shift from "unwell" to "radiant health," we need to address all four.

What's Happening Now	**What's in the Way**	**How You Want to Feel**
Irregular periods Low libido or painful sex Pelvic pain	Gap in Research	Thriving Flourishing Radiant
Hot flashes and night sweats Fertility concerns Adrenal and thyroid dysfunction	Gap in Knowledge	Energized Balanced Powerful Calm
Bloating or other gut problems Difficulty concentrating Anxiety, depression, or irritability	Gap in Care	Focused Resilient Pain-free The best version of you
Sleep disturbances Weight changes Unhealthy skin, hair, or nails	Gap in Confidence	

Gap in Research

Historically, most clinical research has been conducted on men, not women. Until recently, women of childbearing age were excluded from most medical studies. (I share a great deal more about this in Chapter 1.) As a result, we know a lot more about men's bodies than we do about women's, which contributes to a. . .

Gap in Knowledge

In the United States, medical doctors (MDs) and other medical professionals, such as physician assistants (PAs) and nurse practitioners (NPs), receive basic training in how the endocrine system, which controls hormone production, works. However, unless they specialize in endocrinology, their training in this area is limited, especially when it comes to women's hormonal health conditions and care. Gynecologists aren't routinely assessing for generalized hormone-related concerns, and most endocrinologists are seeing patients only once a more advanced endocrine workup or diagnosis is required.

Even physicians who graduate from naturopathic medical school, as I did, don't always receive extensive training in the endocrine system. I chose to specialize in women's health and endocrinology during my postgraduate residencies, fellowships, and research, but not all NDs do. The deeper I went into this field, the more I thought to myself, *I wish every provider had more knowledge in this area, because hormones impact every system in the body, and more women should be screened and supported in the early stages of dysfunction. This is the ultimate in preventative health and wellness.*

Hormones are woven throughout everything, like the invisible fungal mycelium network spreading among vast areas of soil. Once you see how critical hormones are, and all the different roles they perform, you can't unsee it.

In my opinion, failing to empower healthcare professionals with more knowledge about the endocrine system, and women's hormones in particular, is a glaring oversight in our educational system. It disadvantages both medical professionals and their patients. Hormones impact everything from bone density to sleep cycles to metabolism to mood and beyond and, therefore, should be given far more attention in medical training. We know there has been a massive oversight when it comes to menopause, but women's hormones across the entire lifespan still receive far too little attention both in medical training and in patient support.

Because of these educational gaps and the lack of research on women's hormonal health conditions, many medical professionals aren't discussing with their patients how hormones impact every system in the body. Although they have the best of intentions, general primary care providers typically don't run lab tests to check hormone levels, except when it comes to infertility, severe menopause symptoms, or more extreme presentations.

I don't say this to be disparaging toward my colleagues. I encourage every woman to have a primary care provider on her wellness team as well as a gynecologist (GYN). That said, I've heard from countless patients who come to me saying, "My doctor never mentioned that a hormone imbalance could be part of the reason why I don't feel well. . . ." It never came up in conversation.

Just as many providers have knowledge gaps, many women do too. Most women are in the dark, lacking what I consider to be the most basic knowledge about their own bodies. When providers and patients lack information, this creates a. . .

Gap in Care

In an ideal world, every woman would have a complete wellness team, which might include a primary care provider, naturopathic doctor, gynecologist, health coach, therapist, and others, depending on need. Ideally, all these providers would communicate with one another, creating a connected wellness plan rather than a fragmented one.

In the real world, this rarely (if ever) happens. Instead, providers are siloed in their individual specialty areas. Whole body care is generally handled by a woman's primary care provider (PCP) or her GYN. She may then be referred to various specialists as needed. However, these providers rarely collaborate on a well-rounded plan. Appointments are typically too short, nowhere near enough time to get the complete picture of what's going on. And, treatments are far too often pharmaceutical-oriented only, without lifestyle or dietary discussion or preventative wellness strategies.

In our current healthcare system, care tends to be reactive rather than preventative. Symptoms are managed somewhat, but reducing the severity of an uncomfortable symptom is not the same as achieving optimal health.

Although most providers sincerely want to help and are wonderful, kind, intelligent people, they operate within a healthcare system that makes it challenging to provide the care that women need. Strict insurance regulations, understaffing challenges, too many patients, not enough time, and a high level of healthcare provider burnout make it difficult to care for women as whole human beings.

And so, millions of women receive lackluster support. Concerns get dismissed. Issues get misdiagnosed and go untreated.

I can't tell you the number of times I've heard a woman say, "I went to my doctor, described my symptoms, and asked if they could test my hormone levels because I have a strong suspicion that something isn't right. They did the tests, said 'everything looks normal' and offered me a prescription for antidepressants."

What isn't being discussed (on the medical training or patient care side) is that, when it comes to hormone levels, there is a big difference between the "normal" and "optimal" ranges. Normal doesn't necessarily equate to flourishing health. What's more, many don't know that identifying the underlying hormonal issues may require multiple rounds of lab testing, at specific times during a woman's cycle, and particular times of day, and that it's rarely a "one and done" conversation.

Poor-quality care adds to the negative snowball, and over time, this creates a. . .

Gap in Confidence

For centuries, women have been told, "Stop being hysterical." "Don't overreact." "You're fine." "Painful periods? Welcome to being a woman! That's just how it is." "You want to do tests to check your hormone levels? That seems overboard and unnecessary." "It's all just in your head. There's nothing going on with your body."

All this medical gaslighting leads to a situation where women don't trust themselves anymore.

"Maybe I am being dramatic?" she begins to wonder. "Maybe this is normal? Maybe my doctor is right?"

Over time, there is an erosion of confidence. She becomes reluctant to speak up. She has been dismissed before and doesn't want to feel that way again. She begins to lose hope that things can get better. As hope dwindles, she advocates for herself less and less, because what's the point?

The cracks in research, knowledge, care, and confidence compound one another, creating the unfortunate situation that Claudia and so many of my patients are in.

As my colleague Dr. Sara Szal Gottfried puts it, **"It's a health hazard to be female."**

But it shouldn't be, and it doesn't have to be.

Health = Power

I have dedicated my career to solving the hormone-related issues that keep women sick, in pain, or uncomfortable in their bodies and unable to enjoy life to the fullest.

I believe that health is power. It gives you resilience and strength and allows you to live an inspired, abundant life. When you feel good, you can show up without restraint, as your most abundant, shining self. Being in a state of optimal health means you can offer the very best version of yourself to the people you love and the endeavors you care about. Raising children, building a beautiful home, advancing in your career, volunteering, mentoring, writing, creating art, social justice and activism work—you can do everything more powerfully when you are *well*.

Governments, researchers, and medical providers all play a role in improving healthcare outcomes for women. Individual women do, too. We have to take charge and close the gaps that others can't or won't. This means educating ourselves about our bodies, our hormones, and our healthcare options (both allopathic and naturopathic), and being more assertive about our health. Asking questions, rather than automatically saying "yes" to the first treatment plan or prescription that is offered. Doing our own research and leading the conversation, rather than being silent, passive, or intimidated at the doctor's office. This proactive, confident energy is what's needed to improve your own health and to help create the larger societal shifts that we need.

Empowering women to take charge of their lives is one of the main reasons why I felt drawn to a career in healthcare.

My Journey into Medicine

My journey to becoming a naturopathic doctor was an unexpected one. In my 20s, I was leading mountaineering and rock-climbing trips and traveling around the world. I was strong, adventurous, and thriving. But one trip changed everything.

While traveling overseas, I came down with a classic case of traveler's diarrhea. This unpleasant episode led to gastrointestinal dysbiosis, an imbalance in my gut microbiome where the beneficial bacteria become outnumbered by harmful ones. Because I didn't know how to restore my gut microbiome to its ideal state, the imbalance persisted long after my trip ended. Eventually, this snowballed into years of confusing symptoms. Ongoing gut issues. Huge energy crashes. Chronic infections. Hair loss. Anxiety. It was baffling because I led a very healthy lifestyle. I was eating well, exercising, and doing everything "right." Yet, my body kept insisting that something was not okay.

That's when I found naturopathic medicine. Hoping to find answers, I made an appointment. This was the first time a provider looked at *everything*: my gut health, how I handled stress, my hormone levels, my history, and wove it all together. This made all the difference.

It was the first time in my life that I felt a healthcare provider saw *all* of me as part of the solution. Through natural, personalized treatment and true whole-body healthcare, I began to heal. Within a year, I felt more vibrant and healthier than ever, even before I had become sick.

This experience changed everything for me, and it's why I became a naturopathic doctor myself. I see so many patients now who are in that same place, feeling unwell, without answers, despite their best efforts, and despite seeing all the specialists.

What Is Naturopathic Medicine?

When I introduce myself as a naturopathic doctor, many don't know what this means. The word *naturopathic* might conjure up images of burning incense, chanting around a fire pit, or vials filled with mysterious potions. Not exactly.

Naturopathic medicine is regulated by federal accreditation and state licensing boards. To become a licensed naturopathic doctor (ND), also referred to as a naturopathic physician or naturopathic medical doctor (NMD), you must graduate from an accredited four-year medical school program and pass multiple rigorous licensing exams. Like an MD, our required exams include a Part I: Biomedical Science (covering anatomy, physiology, pathology, and biochemistry) and Part II: Core Clinical Science (clinical sciences, diagnosis, and treatment modalities specific to naturopathic medicine, such as pharmacology, nutrition, and botanical medicine), as well as some elective state-specific jurisprudence exams.

Naturopathic medical students study both biomedical sciences and naturopathic and conventional therapeutics, including anatomy, physiology, biochemistry, pathology, pharmacology, botanical medicine, clinical nutrition, physical medicine, hydrotherapy, IV therapy, and minor surgery. Our education incorporates the latest advances in science and natural approaches to illness prevention and management. Students complete a minimum of 4,100 hours of class and clinical training, including more than 1,200 hours of hands-on, supervised clinical training.

Upon gaining licensure, naturopathic doctors can order diagnostic tests such as blood tests, X-rays, and MRIs; diagnose diseases, do injectable or IV therapy; prescribe prescription drugs (including hormone replacement therapy [HRT]); and perform certain types of minor surgery.

I share this information to reassure you that this book is grounded in scientific evidence. Naturopathic doctors are real doctors, just like medical doctors. The difference is that we take different approaches in our work.

As a naturopathic doctor, I use the least invasive therapies (including lifestyle and dietary adjustments, botanical medicine, and targeted nutrient, amino acid, and hormone therapy) first and then move on to more invasive therapies (like medications and surgery) only as a last resort. I focus on resolving the root cause of my patient's distress, rather than masking symptoms to create temporary relief. And when a woman describes her symptoms, even very minor ones, I see it as part of the bigger picture. Small, subtle symptoms are often a clue as to what's really going on. The approach is truly the deepest form of whole-body preventive wellness, with the goal of maximizing *health span*, not just lifespan.

You might see your primary care provider (PCP) once a year for an annual check-up or when you have an acute concern, and more often when you have a chronic one. NDs automatically work more intensively with every patient. We typically have longer, more frequent appointments—monthly or every couple of months—for six months to a year, because creating profound change takes time and requires truly knowing someone's story and understanding their patterns.

Conventional medicine saves countless lives. If you have a broken leg, are bleeding profusely, are experiencing a stroke, or have an infection, or your life is in immediate peril for any reason, this is when you should absolutely see a conventional provider. Go to the hospital and see an MD or a specialist, because they have the skills to help.

But conventional medicine, in the form that is most practiced today, is not a complete solution. If you are dealing with an issue that is vague, mysterious, subtle, complicated, multifaceted (its origin is emotional, mental, and physical), not life-threatening but still unpleasant, or chronic and ongoing, or simply wanting to incorporate more natural medicine modalities, nutrition, lifestyle, botanical medicine, etc., naturopathic medicine may be a better fit. Both forms of medicine are powerful and have their place and can be used together.

Naturopathic Doctors Versus Naturopaths

Lastly, I want to mention that "naturopaths" and "naturopathic doctors" are not the same thing. You may occasionally see someone refer to themself as a "naturopath." Generally, this person is an unlicensed practitioner who did not attend medical school. They might be gifted healers in spiritual or emotional coaching, energy healing, ancient rituals involving plant medicine, and so on, but they are not licensed doctors. Be mindful of this when choosing which providers to bring onto your wellness team. (Note: after the book's conclusion, I provide a glossary that defines important terms to know, including a list of healthcare professionals—medical doctors, naturopathic doctors, nurse practitioners, phlebotomists, midwives, and more—if you are interested in learning more about what each of these providers do, their similarities, and differences.)

My Training and Credentials

After experiencing the power of naturopathic medicine firsthand and seeing how dramatically it transformed my body and life, I felt called to practice it myself. I was honored to be accepted to one of the top naturopathic schools in the world, began my studies, and went all in.

After graduating from the National University of Natural Medicine (NUNM) with my doctorate, I completed a highly selective postdoctoral women's health residency. This residency included two years of fellowship rotations in conventional gynecology and endocrinology (general and reproductive), as well as mentorship from one of the leading pioneers in naturopathic women's medicine, with a specific focus on menopause care.

I also completed a two-year research fellowship with the School of Research and Graduate Studies at the Helfgott Research Institute. As a researcher, I investigated topics such as preconception, infertility, HPV/cervical dysplasia, gastrointestinal health, and interstitial cystitis, and published in numerous medical journals. My research fellowship was followed by an adjunct faculty position at NUNM, the same university where I earned my doctorate.

By this point in my story, I was a mom of two, and my husband and I wanted to live closer to our parents so the girls could see their grandparents regularly. The only problem was that my parents lived on the West Coast, while my husband's were on the East Coast. After a great deal of deliberation, weighing all the pros and cons, we decided to move east. That's when I opened my own practice as a licensed naturopathic doctor in Portland, Maine.

My practice, Naturopathic by Design®, is a women's health clinic that now employs a team of naturopathic doctors like myself, along with registered nurses, phlebotomists, functional health coaches, nutritionists, midwives, and more.

Today, I hold a doctor of naturopathic medicine, a master of science in integrative medicine research, and a bachelor of arts with an emphasis in medical anthropology. I have been published in medical journals, including *Integrative Medicine: A Clinician's Journal*, *Explore: The Journal of Science and Healing*, *Journal of Ayurveda and Integrative Medicine*, *Mental Health & Prevention*, and others. In addition to running my clinic, I've been invited to serve as a consultant and medical advisor for natural health companies such as LOLA (menstrual and sexual wellness products) and Beeya Wellness (organic superfoods to support hormonal balance).

I am known for bridging the divide between conventional and natural medicine, bringing together evidence-based science with naturopathic approaches.

Every woman who steps into my practice is unique. But I have noticed a common thread: a deep knowing that something is off and that things could be better.

Many of my clients have never experienced naturopathic medicine before—and once they do, it's the missing piece they have been searching for.

Changing the Trajectory

We often think of care as either preventative or reactive, but *real healing doesn't live in either extreme*. It lives in the space between, and in the layers and nuances, where you stop the negative snowball effect and change the trajectory.

Like nudging the nose of an airplane just a few degrees mid-flight, small course corrections can mean the difference between crashing and arriving safely home.

That's what this book offers:

A course correction
A way back to your own body
A path to reclaim your power

What's Ahead

Throughout *Hormone Powered*, you'll learn:

- All about hormones: the chemical messengers that transport signals all around your body
- How hormones impact not just your menstrual cycle but *everything* in your body—your digestion, energy levels, ability to fight off diseases, and beyond

- What happens when hormone levels are too low, too high, and just right
- The root causes of your symptoms, even the "mystery" ones
- Which lab tests are worth doing and how to interpret your results
- The three primary Hormone Types that I see in my practice, an assessment to figure out which type you are, and what it may mean about your health
- How to support your hormones (with or without medication) so you can feel the best you can possibly feel
- How to build your own custom wellness plan—which I call your *Hormone Action Plan*—that is grounded in evidence and extremely effective

Reclaiming Your Power

Imagine your healthiest, most vibrant self, standing a mile away. So far, you can barely even see her. Such a big distance between your current self and the self you want to be.

But as you move through this book, you'll learn how to start closing the gap. A mile will become a half mile, then a quarter mile, then just a few feet. Eventually, no separation at all.

It may take time to close the gap. It did for Claudia, the client I mentioned earlier who was in a state of tremendous distress.

With Claudia, we decided to go back to basics and zoom out to examine her whole-body health: early menstrual history, habits, nutrition, and side-effect profiles of her medications. We checked her nutrient levels, corrected her iron and other vitamin deficiencies, and addressed her stimulant habit. We got her started on a sufficient dose of body-identical (bio-identical) hormone therapy to support what her body could no longer make. We got her sleeping, moving, and building momentum as she watched her body change. Then, as we gradually reduced her psychiatric medications, she noticed a significant change, like a long-term suppressive fog lifting or signs of spring after a long, dark winter. Slowly but surely, the vibrant person she truly is began to shine through.

Though it took several adjustments to her diet, lifestyle, and natural medicine helpers, addressing her nutrient deficiencies was crucial in her recovery and to her mental health recovery.

It took time, but the momentum of the work instilled an internal sense of truly knowing what was possible that kept her going. She eventually came off all her medication and regained control over her sleep, energy, and mood. Her passions began to shine through, and she started to dream of all the possibilities ahead in her life. She also began a new romantic relationship rooted in support and care and made exciting changes in her career.

What happened wasn't magic. It was physiology. It was whole-body hormone care. And it was long overdue.

If a woman like Claudia can return to a state of flourishing health—even after years of physical and emotional anguish that was so severe, she wasn't sure she wanted to exist anymore—I know it is possible for you, too.

As a doctor, researcher, and mother, I stand in the center of conventional and naturopathic medicine. Not on one extreme end or the other but in the middle. Translating. Integrating. Fighting for nuance. And helping women find answers.

So, if you're one of those women who thinks, "I know I could feel a lot better than I currently do," this book is for you.

Your body is not the problem. The system is.

The situation is not hopeless. You have more options than you might realize.

Once you understand how to take better care of your hormones, the sacred chemical messengers that influence every system in your body, and keep them balanced, you will be amazed by what a difference you see and feel.

As many of my patients say, "I feel like the lights are back on. I have come back to life."

Let's reclaim your power—together.

How to Use This Book

"What brings you in today?"

It's the first question I ask a new patient.

Although we may be thousands of miles apart, this book is a conversation between you and me.

So, I'd like to begin by asking you that same question: what brought you here?

If you're like many of my patients, you might be experiencing frustrating symptoms (painful, irregular, or missing periods, bloating and digestive issues, skin breakouts, hair loss, weight changes, premenstrual syndrome (PMS) and premenstrual dysphoric disorder (PMDD), low libido, anxiety, depression, fatigue, brain fog, trouble focusing, insomnia, migraines, fertility or perimenopausal struggles, and more) and are longing for relief.

Or you might be someone who feels pretty good overall. No major symptoms are bothering you. Yet, you suspect you could be feeling better than you currently do. You want to shift from feeling "okay" or "good" to "incredible."

Perhaps you're aware that a big hormonal shift, like perimenopause or menopause, is right around the corner. You want to learn about your body so that you can have a smooth transition into this next phase. You'd like to avoid the hormonal drama and discomfort that you've heard other women talking about!

Whatever brought you here, welcome, and thank you.

The following is an overview of how this book is structured and how to get the best possible results.

Part One: Know Your Body

Most women have limited knowledge about the important functions that hormones perform because they were never taught any of this. In Part One, you'll receive the foundational education you need.

You'll learn what hormones are (there are more than 50 hormones in your body, and each one plays a vital role), what they do, how they communicate with one another, and what happens when certain hormone levels are too high, too low, or just right.

Part Two: Find Out Your Type

After reading Part One, you'll understand the basics about women's hormones and what they do. Your next step is to complete an online assessment to find out your primary Hormone Type.

You'll answer a series of questions about your health history, recurring patterns you notice in your life, symptoms you tend to experience, and more.

This assessment is free, and you can find it here:

Scan or visit https://drcorinadunlap.com/assessment/.

After serving thousands of patients during my postdoctoral residencies and fellowships and at the women's health clinic that I run today, I have noticed that most women fall into one of three categories when it comes to their hormonal health. I call these three categories Hormone Types.

The three types are the Caretaker, the Achiever, and the Survivor. In Part Two, you'll find a chapter dedicated to each type, where I share what's happening at the biomedical level for each.

Once you know your Hormone Type, you can design a wellness plan that's highly effective for you—a plan that is personalized, not generic.

Part Three: Create Your Hormone Action Plan

Next, it's time to create your personalized wellness plan. I call this your Hormone Action Plan.

This is the plan that will take you from feeling "terrible" to "okay" to "good" to eventually "fantastic."

In Part Three, you will learn about the seven components of your Hormone Action Plan and how to tailor your plan to your Hormone Type.

Build Your Team—and Lead the Conversation

At the center of a successful wellness plan is your support network. This can include friends and family who want to see you thrive, as well as healthcare providers like your naturopathic doctor, medical doctor, obstetrician-gynecologist, nurse practitioner, and others.

I don't recommend implementing your Hormone Action Plan on your own. I *do* recommend discussing your plan with licensed professionals whom you trust. Think of *Hormone Powered* as a playbook that you're using in collaboration with the professionals on your support team.

This book + you + licensed healthcare professionals =
a winning formula.

Hormone Powered isn't meant to replace your provider. It's meant to empower you before you even walk in the door for your next appointment. Too often, women go to the doctor feeling overwhelmed and confused and then say "okay" to the first solution proposed to them, which may or may not be effective. What I want is for you to visit your provider and *lead* the conversation, rather than going along with whatever they suggest.

Optional, but Recommended: Do Lab Testing

In addition to reading this book and implementing what you have learned, I encourage you to do lab testing not only to check your hormone levels but also to get a more complete picture of what can contribute to hormone health. This step is optional but highly recommended.

Why do this? If you're noticing distressing symptoms of any kind—weight gain, fatigue, skin issues, stomach problems, and beyond—most likely something is off with one (or more) of the 50 different hormones in your body. Certain levels might be too high or too low. You might have deficiencies that can lead to hormone-related diseases and illnesses.

Based on the symptoms you're experiencing, it's possible for you (or your healthcare provider) to take an educated guess as to which hormones are out of balance. But the only way to know for sure is through lab testing. As I often say to my patients, "I'm a big fan of testing, rather than guessing."

I created a Lab Testing Guide for you. It's online, free, and you can access it here:

Scan or visit www.drcorinadunlap.com/labtestingguide/

This guide includes:

- A checklist of the top lab tests that I recommend doing
- Ideal timing to do each test (some tests should be done first thing in the morning on an empty stomach, others are best done at specific points in your menstrual cycle, etc.)
- How to order these labs yourself, even if you get pushback from a provider
- How to make sense of your testing results, including understanding the difference between "normal" levels versus "optimal"

Most of the lab tests that I recommend are done with a blood or saliva sample. Some may be covered by your insurance, depending on various factors.

I recommend doing all (or as many as possible) of the tests listed in the Lab Testing Guide. This will give you a complete picture of where you are now. In the future, you can test again to see how your levels have changed.

Implement Your Plan—Then Do Follow-Up Testing

After starting your Hormone Action Plan, follow up with lab testing three months later to see how your levels have changed.

(In certain cases, such as a thyroid dysfunction, you may want to do follow-up testing sooner than three months. Discuss this with your provider.)

If your plan is working, you should see exciting changes in your lab reports after about three months. Hormones should return to optimal ranges rather than remain too low or too high. You should notice physiological and emotional changes, too: acne clearing, hair growth improving, GI issues resolving, energy levels increasing, brain fog clearing, and so on. Positive signs of progress!

If your follow-up testing doesn't show much improvement in your levels or you are not feeling better, this is your sign to tweak your wellness plan to get things moving in the right direction. You may need to tweak your diet, sleep habits, stress management, or something else, depending on your situation. There may also be something deeper going on. (More on this in Part Three.) Again, working with a naturopathic doctor or another provider can help you fine-tune your plan to get it dialed in exactly where it needs to be. Remember the winning formula: this book + you + your support team = radiant health. Support is everything. You don't have to walk this path alone.

Those are my suggestions for getting the best possible results from this book. To sum it up briefly:

1. Read the book.
2. Use my guidance to create your Hormone Action Plan.
3. Put your plan into action.
4. Conduct lab testing to assess how effectively your plan is working.

Regain Your Power—One Small Step at a Time

If you are feeling a bit overwhelmed right now ("I have so much to learn, so many tests to do, so many changes to make. . ."), take a big, deep breath. Know this: you don't have to do lab testing today.

Or find a new provider. Or check your health insurance coverage info. Or overhaul your entire lifestyle. For now, you can inhale, exhale, and turn the page. Take things slowly, one step at a time.

I'll leave you with these encouraging words:

Sometimes, the changes that make the most significant difference for your health are very small and so doable. Going to bed a bit earlier. Taking a screen-free morning. Tweaking your diet just a little bit by anchoring each meal with protein. All these micro-changes impact your hormones, and the changes accumulate and create momentum. Eventually, the negative snowball effect of hormone dysregulation reverses and becomes a positive one.

Your body was designed to flourish and thrive.

You can get back to that place, and it will happen one step at a time.

I'm here with you, through every step. I hope that *Hormone Powered* becomes a treasured addition to your bookshelf and a guide that you return to for many years to come.

—Dr. Corina Dunlap

Note on Names and Pronouns

Throughout the book, you will hear a few stories about my patients. I share these stories to illustrate medical concepts more clearly, to help readers feel less alone in their struggles, and to provide hope that change is possible.

Patient names and other identifying details (such as the woman's profession or location) have been changed for privacy, while preserving the essence and truth of the narrative.

Although I primarily use words like "woman," "she," and "her" in my writing, I want to acknowledge that some people who have a female reproductive system, and who are assigned female at birth, do not identify as women. For this reason, I occasionally use terms like "they" and "them" to be inclusive of all gender identities.

Whether you personally identify as female, nonbinary, or another identity, I hope you will feel seen in these pages—and that the guidance I provide helps you feel vibrant, healthy, and at home in your body.

Part One

KNOW YOUR BODY

When I was a teenager, my high school offered very rudimentary lessons on health, wellness, and reproductive topics.

The "education" (and that's a generous term!) provided to us was extremely simplistic.

The gist of it was:

- "Girls, at some point, if it hasn't already happened, your body will change, and you will get your period."
- "Right before your period, you might feel irritable, feel sad, have cramps, or feel bloated. You can blame hormones for that! Take some Midol."
- "Hormones cause you to feel emotional and make risky choices, like having sex."
- "If you have unprotected sex, you may get pregnant. You could also catch an STI. Practice abstinence or use a condom."

And that was pretty much the extent of it. Extremely little info. Very basic. No nuance. Hormones were mentioned, but only briefly, and the emphasis was that "hormones make you feel crappy" or compel you to make "bad choices." Almost as though they are negative, even sinister.

As a result, like millions of women, I grew up with very little information about my own body, mystified and in the dark. It wasn't until much later in life that I got the education I should have had all along.

Poor Education, Poor Outcomes

Here in the United States, we do not have a unified, integrated approach to teaching health, wellness, and reproductive topics in public schools. Some schools don't cover it at all.

As of 2024, only 30 out of 50 U.S. states have laws requiring that sex education be taught in schools, though these laws do not necessarily ensure a thorough or high-quality education.[1] Even when these topics are covered, the curriculum is often perfunctory at best. Students are given the tip of the iceberg, if that. So much gets missed.

Only five states require comprehensive sex education (CSE), a higher standard of education that, as defined by the World Health Organization, can include "life skills," "families and relationships," "respect, consent and bodily autonomy," "anatomy, puberty, and menstruation," and "contraception and pregnancy," among other topics.[2]

My point being: if your high school covered these topics at all—which isn't a given—it's unlikely they were covered with any nuance.

Unfortunately, after high school, as you step into adulthood, you're likely to encounter more of the same. When visiting your doctor, even if they would love to educate you about your body, they usually don't have time to do it. Quick appointments, scheduled back-to-back, with little to no buffer space in between, aren't conducive to lengthy, thoughtful discussions about your health.

It's not that doctors don't *want* to educate their patients—most of them do, and many of them try very hard to fit it in—but the systems and scheduling realities of conventional medicine make it difficult to talk about anything in depth.

In the United States, we have worse health outcomes, higher rates of many chronic diseases, and lower life expectancy compared to many high-income economies. This is unsurprising, because if we have glaring educational gaps and don't really understand how our bodies work in the first place, how can we possibly take good care of ourselves? We are fumbling around in the fog, gathering scraps of information (which may or may not be accurate) from social media influencers, podcasters, or clickbait news headlines ("Do This One Hormone Trick to Instantly Melt Belly Fat and Look 20 Years Younger!"). There's so much health-related content out there, much of it contradictory, and it can feel overwhelming to make sense of it all.

Part One: Know Your Body is my attempt to cut through the confusion by providing the education that you should have received decades ago—but probably didn't.

I will cover what hormones are, some of the most important ones to know about, and the roles they play in your body.

You'll learn about your endocrine system, which produces and regulates hormones, and how it is supposed to evolve throughout the seasons of your life: puberty, pregnancy, postpartum, perimenopause, menopause, and beyond.

I'll explain how your hormones communicate with one another, what happens when the conversation gets disrupted, and when certain hormone levels get too high or too low.

My hope is that, after reading Part One, you will feel informed and in awe of your body.

Knowledge is power, especially when it comes to your health and hormones.

Even if high school was a long time ago, it's never too late to get empowered.

Notes

1. "Detailed Insights on U.S. Sex Education Policies." Sexuality Information and Education Council of the United States. SIECUS. 2024. https://siecus.org/state-profiles-2024/.
2. "Comprehensive Sexuality Education." World Health Organization. WHO. 2023. https://www.who.int/news-room/questions-and-answers/item/comprehensive-sexuality-education.

Chapter 1

Hormones: Your Body's Mighty Messengers

You are not behind.

I know this for a fact—and as a doctor and researcher, I don't use that word lightly.

How do I know this? Because for the past 10 years, I've been an adjunct faculty member at a top school of graduate studies. My students are among the brightest minds in the medical field and are completing their doctorates.

Every time I begin my class on female fertility, I give them a pop quiz.

I ask my students to pull out a blank piece of paper and draw the menstrual cycle.

"I want you to label each phase of the cycle," I instruct them. "Write down the main hormones involved in each phase and what each hormone does—not only in the uterus but across the whole body."

You know what I get? Blank stares. Awkward silence. Maybe a half-hearted diagram or two. But very few have a solid grasp of what I believe should be foundational education for every adolescent, and certainly every healthcare provider. This is Human Physiology 101!

No medical student wants to be caught unprepared. I probably don't make the most popular first impression on my new students, but I make one they won't forget.

The point of the exercise is simple and powerful: if you're going to care for people—especially women—you need to understand not just how life *begins* but how it *sustains*.

And that's how I know: you are not behind.

You are not behind for not understanding the basics of your own cycle.

You are not behind for not knowing what your hormones are doing or what hormones even *are* in the first place.

You are not behind.

You have been failed by a system that doesn't teach this information, not even to most medical professionals.

Missing the Basics

When healthcare providers lack even the most basic understanding of women's hormones, they can't possibly serve women at the level they need and deserve. When women lack this information, too, they can't advocate for themselves at the doctor's office or even know which questions to ask.

There is a knowledge gap on both sides—provider and patient—and this creates a negative ripple effect. The knowledge gap results in a dangerous care gap, and women are the ones who pay the price.

Longer Lives, but Poorer Quality

Statistically, women live longer than men but spend 25% more of their lives in poorer health.[1] This is what researchers call a "morbidity disadvantage."

Many chronic illnesses, including the ones that aren't fatal but negatively affect your quality of life, can be traced back to hormonal imbalances. Hormones shape immunity, metabolism, pain perception, cardiovascular function, neurological patterns, and how women respond to medications, yet hormonal dynamics have been minimized or misunderstood for decades. Diseases that disproportionately affect women, including endometriosis, polyendocrine metabolic ovarian syndrome (PMOS), chronic pain conditions, autoimmune disorders, and many mood disorders, have been underfunded, under-researched, and often dismissed as "complex" or "too variable" to study. The result is a persistent, systemic blind spot: a health landscape where women are living longer but living sicker, not because their bodies are inherently flawed but because the science meant to support them never kept pace with their needs.

Despite the enormous influence that hormones have on our well-being, they are deeply misunderstood, even in medical communities.

Why We Know So Little About Women's Bodies

Why are so many women in poor health? And why are hormonal issues chronically underdiagnosed and undertreated?[2]

One of the biggest reasons is lack of research. Until recently, women were excluded from most medical research trials. Why? Primarily to avoid harming unborn fetuses from testing that might lead to birth defects. In 1977, the Food & Drug Administration (FDA) issued a policy advising researchers to avoid doing testing on "women of childbearing potential." As journalist Maya Dusenbery explains in her award-winning book *Doing Harm: The Truth About How Bad Medicine and Lazy Science Leave Women Dismissed, Misdiagnosed, and Sick*,[3] this effectively meant all women of reproductive age were excluded, regardless of whether they intended to have children or not, setting women's health research back by decades.

This policy was problematic for many reasons, the most obvious being that it presumes that every woman *wants* to have children or have *more* children. And the policy had unintended consequences. Whenever a new procedure or medication hit the market, it had been tested on men, but not women. Dusenbery documents how these policies have had real, life-threatening consequences: drugs withdrawn in the late 1990s were nearly twice as likely to cause harm in women, simply because no one had tested for sex differences in metabolism, side effects, or dosage.

To quote journalist Olivia Cassano, "Much of modern medicine is based on research done exclusively on male bodies, and the consequences of this research gap are significant—sometimes even life-threatening."[4]

But avoiding the possibility of harming unborn children isn't the only reason why women have been excluded from research. In the past, women's hormonal fluctuations were deemed "too complicated" for many studies. Including women as test subjects would mean additional nuances to consider (and additional costs) that researchers didn't want to take on. As Dusenbery notes in *Doing Harm*, women were often perceived as "outliers" who might skew study results, rather than what they actually are: more than half of the world's population. For all these reasons—cost, complexity, gender biases in the medical community—women were pushed out of studies that ought to have placed them right in the center.

Then in 1993, things changed, at least, somewhat. That's when the U.S. National Institutes of Health (NIH) released the Revitalization Act,[5] which made it mandatory to include women in clinical trials funded by the NIH, unless a clear and compelling reason for exclusion could be provided. Although this act was a step in the right direction, it wasn't a miracle fix, for two major reasons. One, not all trials are funded by the NIH. Two, because women were excluded from research for so many decades, this created a cumulative effect, a research deficiency that is so large it will take many more decades to close it. Even after some policies were lifted, the inertia of exclusion had already shaped the healthcare field. In short, we still have a lot of catching up to do.

And so, what we have today is a massive void in clinical knowledge. Even now, women's hormonal concerns often fall outside of conventional diagnostic models and treatment protocols. If it doesn't fit neatly into a box, many doctors don't know what to do with it. Hence, that is why so many women get turned away when they ask to have their hormones tested. Most doctors don't even know the basics of what they would be testing for, the appropriate timing of the cycle, or what to do with the results.

Because of this gap in research and the resulting scarcity in knowledge, when women describe distressing symptoms, they often get dismissed. I've had countless patients who go to their doctor's office and describe frustrating issues: weight gain, fatigue, low libido, skin issues, depression, anxiety, and beyond, and they are told, "Everything on your lab report looks normal." "I'm not seeing anything that looks concerning." Or, "Welcome to being in your 40s!"

If the patient pushes further, insisting that something just isn't right, they are often told, "Let's keep an eye on things" (which essentially means, "Come back and see me if things get really, really bad, so bad that you're no longer able to function"). In the meantime, they are offered a birth control prescription or antidepressants and sent on their way.

Let's call this what it is: *medical gaslighting*. This is when a healthcare provider dismisses or downplays a patient's concerns, minimizing, brushing aside, or invalidating a woman's experience. This doesn't happen on purpose or because the provider doesn't care; most do. It happens because of a lack of knowledge that leaves both patients and providers in the dark.

This is why millions of women are told:

- "There is nothing wrong." (Even when they *know* deep down this is not the case.)

- "What you're experiencing is normal." (Just because something is common doesn't mean it's okay.)
- "You need to wait until you are in severe distress, so severe that you are nonfunctional, and only *then* will medical professionals leap into action to help you." (This part is unspoken but implied through a provider's inaction.)

All this dismissal chips away at our confidence. We question ourselves and wonder, "Maybe they are right? Maybe this is just what it means to be a woman? Maybe feeling 'not great' is normal? Perhaps this really is as good as it gets?"

Education Is the First Step

What is the solution? How can we create a better world—a world in which women's pain is taken seriously, conditions are diagnosed and treated appropriately, and women spend most of their lives in excellent health?

The first step is to educate yourself about your own body. You need to understand what hormones are, how they communicate with one another, and how they impact your well-being.

It's challenging to choose the right healthcare provider, get your concerns taken seriously, and collaborate with your wellness team successfully, when you don't have the knowledge (or language) to describe what's going on.

Starting now? We're going to change that.

You have probably heard the term *financial literacy*. That's the idea that every human being needs a basic understanding of how to earn, spend, save, and invest for the future. Everyone needs money to navigate the world; therefore, this information should be in everyone's hands—not just professional financial advisors!

The same is true when it comes to your body. We need *hormone literacy*, too.

Every woman should know the information we're about to cover. My hope is that you'll take this in, feel more empowered, and one day pass the info along to a young woman in your life.

What Are Hormones?

Hormones are the mighty messengers of your body. They are chemical signals that travel through your bloodstream and lymph fluid, delivering instructions to organs and tissues to help keep everything running smoothly.

Your hormones influence nearly every aspect of your health—not just your menstrual cycle, sexual health, and reproduction. Your metabolism, sleep, energy levels, mood, brain function, muscle health, bone density—hormones impact all of these.

When hormones are in balance and communicating properly, your body thrives. You feel vibrant. You flourish. You feel like "your best self."

But if they are too low, too high, or miscommunicating, you feel it. When there is a disturbance in the network, your body starts speaking to you through symptoms. At first, whispering. Later, shouting.

These symptoms are not a punishment, they're a signal. This is your body's way of saying, "Help, please! Something is not right. Please pay attention to me. . .."

Meet the Endocrine System

You might be familiar with some of the major systems in your body. For instance, your digestive system breaks down food into fuel and waste. Your cardiovascular system transports oxygen around your body. Your nervous system scans for potential threats in your surroundings and notifies your brain that "it's safe to relax" or "warning, danger!" And your endocrine system controls hormone production.

The endocrine system consists of a network of glands (think: pituitary, thyroid, parathyroid, adrenals, pancreas, ovaries, and in men, testes) that produce and release these mighty messengers.

Your endocrine system produces more than 50 hormones. You don't need to memorize every single one of them. But it's a good idea to get familiar with *some* of them—the key players.

Let's start with the top five you need to know.

Meet the VIHs: Very Important Hormones

The VIPs of the female hormone world (or rather, VIHs) are estrogen, progesterone, testosterone, cortisol, and melatonin. Here's how these hormones impact your body, the role they perform, and what it feels like when they're too low or too high:

Estrogen The *Radiance* Hormone			
Affects	***Role***	***Too Low***	***Too High***
Mood, memory, motivation, metabolism, bones, heart, gut, muscles, skin, and body temperature.	Estrogen energizes your whole body. It balances brain chemicals like serotonin and dopamine, protects your heart and bones, boosts metabolism, and gives your skin, mood, and mind a vibrant, youthful glow. It lights you up from the inside out, giving you a glow of vitality.	Drained energy, dull mood, disrupted sleep, stiffness, and a sense of *slowing down.*	Tension, irritability, headaches, puffiness, and emotional volatility.

Progesterone **The *Calm, Clear Mind* Hormone**			
Affects	***Role***	***Too Low***	***Too High***
Mental clarity, calm, sleep, digestion, immunity, and reproductive balance.	Progesterone supports gamma-aminobutyric acid (GABA), the neurotransmitter that promotes deep sleep, stabilizes mood, protects the brain, soothes digestion, and prepares the body for rest, repair, and reproduction; the hormone of serenity and stability.	Tired, but wired: anxious, restless, sleepless, and emotionally thin.	Calm, but heavy: Fatigue, bloating, slowed digestion, low motivation, and mental dullness.

Testosterone **The *Get It Done!* Hormone**			
Affects	***Role***	***Too Low***	***Too High***
Drive, confidence, assertiveness, motivation, libido, energy, focus, muscle tone, and bone strength.	Testosterone fuels energy, motivation, and confidence. It sharpens focus, builds strength, enhances libido, and gives you the inner spark to take action and feel powerful.	Low energy, low sex drive, less muscle tone, and loss of inner "drive" or spark.	Edgy, impatient, breakout-prone, and overly amped.

Cortisol **The *Stress and Resilience* Hormone**			
Affects	***Role***	***Too Low***	***Too High***
Stress response, stamina, energy, focus, sleep, immunity, metabolism, mood, and inflammation control.	Cortisol is your body's built-in alarm system. It mobilizes energy, sharpens focus, regulates inflammation, and helps you adapt to physical or emotional stress so you can stay alert and survive.	Drained, foggy, easily overwhelmed, and burnt out, unable to rally under stress.	Constantly on, tense, restless, gaining belly weight, with trouble relaxing or sleeping.

Melatonin **The *Rest and Repair* Hormone**			
Affects	***Role***	***Too Low***	***Too High***
Sleep quality, circadian rhythm, cellular repair, immune strength, metabolism, mood, reproduction, and aging.	Melatonin is your body's "darkness signal"—it synchronizes your sleep-wake cycle, triggers nighttime cellular repair, supports immune defense, regulates reproductive hormones, and shields the body from oxidative stress.	Restless nights, brain fog, low immunity, and feeling older or "off rhythm."	Too sleepy, foggy, or emotionally flat and "stuck in nighttime mode."

To recap, estrogen, progesterone, testosterone (yes, women produce this hormone too!), cortisol, and melatonin are five of the most important hormones in your body. If your life were an HBO series, these five are the main characters—the stars of the show. However, there are many other hormones that perform important functions, too.

Two supporting cast members you need to know are triiodothyronine (abbreviated as T3) and thyroxine (aka T4), which are produced by your thyroid gland. They aren't at the center of every episode but still play an important role in the story.

Triiodothyronine (T3) and Thyroxine (T4) **The *Metabolic Duo***			
Affects	***Role***	***Too Low***	***Too High***
Energy, metabolism, mood, menstrual cycles, hair/skin health, temperature regulation.	Thyroid hormones are like your body's thermostat and conductor, setting the pace for how every cell produces energy and how efficiently your body runs.	Fatigue, brain fog, weight gain, hair thinning, constipation, irregular cycles, and feeling cold.	Anxiety, heart palpitations, unintentional weight loss, heat intolerance, and difficulty sleeping.

Now you've been introduced to a few of the most important hormones in your body. But what about all the other hormones? They matter, too.

Let's meet a few more of these chemical messengers.

Additional Hormones to Know

As I mentioned earlier, your body produces more than 50 hormones. Each one has a unique job. While I won't cover all of them in this book, I want to introduce you to some.

Do you need to memorize all of them? No. However, it's a good idea to take a quick glance so you're somewhat familiar with these terms.

Why do this?

One, glancing at this big list of hormones will give you an instant appreciation for how incredible hormones are and all the various things they do. This helps you understand why hormone care needs to be a central focus in your wellness plan, not an afterthought.

And two, because the next time you're meeting with someone on your healthcare team, you'll be more informed about your body. You'll know the names of the various chemical messengers and what they do. You'll have the vocabulary to ask thoughtful questions about your health. Knowledge is power.

In each of the following tables, at the top I state the endocrine gland that produces the hormones beneath it:

Hypothalamus ***Located in the center of the brain***	
Thyrotropin-releasing hormone (TRH)	Triggers the pituitary to release thyroid-stimulating hormone (TSH), which stimulates the thyroid to regulate metabolism, energy, and body temperature
Growth hormone-releasing hormone (GHRH)	Signals the pituitary to release growth hormone (GH), supporting tissue repair, muscle growth, and metabolic function

(continued)

(continued)

Corticotropin-releasing hormone (CRH)	Stimulates the pituitary to release adrenocorticotropic hormone (ACTH), activating the adrenal glands and initiating the stress response
Somatostatin (growth hormone-inhibiting hormone)	Inhibits the release of growth hormone (GH) from the pituitary, helping regulate growth and metabolism
Prolactin-inhibiting hormone (PIH)	Suppresses prolactin release from the pituitary, regulating milk production and reproductive balance

Pituitary Gland (Anterior) ***Located at the base of the brain***	
Luteinizing hormone (LH)	Stimulates ovulation and corpus luteum formation; triggers progesterone production
Follicle-stimulating hormone (FSH)	Stimulates growth of ovarian follicles and estrogen production
Prolactin	Promotes milk production postpartum; can suppress ovulation when elevated
Adrenocorticotropic hormone (ACTH)	Stimulates cortisol production by the adrenals; involved in stress response
Thyroid-stimulating hormone (TSH)	Regulates thyroid hormone production—vital for metabolism and hormonal synergy

Pituitary Gland (Posterior) ***Located at the base of the brain***	
Oxytocin	Released directly into the bloodstream to support childbirth, lactation, and emotional bonding
Vasopressin (antidiuretic hormone, ADH)	Helps regulate hydration and blood pressure by signaling the kidneys to retain water

Pineal Gland ***Located in the center of the brain, in a groove between the two hemispheres***	
Melatonin	Regulates circadian rhythm and influences reproductive hormone secretion (including timing of puberty and cycle regularity)

Ovaries ***Located in the pelvis, on either side of the uterus***	
Estrogen (mainly estradiol, E2)	Drives development of female secondary sex characteristics, endometrial growth, mood, skin, libido, and bone health
Progesterone	Prepares uterine lining for implantation, supports early pregnancy, calms the nervous system, modulates immune response
Testosterone	Supports libido, bone density, muscle mass, motivation, and mood (yes—ovaries make this too!)
Inhibin A & B	Inhibit FSH release; help regulate follicle development and menstrual cycle timing
Anti-Müllerian hormone (AMH)	Reflects ovarian reserve; produced by small growing follicles

Adrenal Glands ***Located at the top of each kidney***	
Cortisol	Regulates stress response, blood sugar, metabolism, and inflammation; impacts cycle regularity and ovulation under chronic stress
DHEA/DHEA-S	Precursor to sex hormones (especially androgens); supports mood, libido, and energy
Adrenaline and noradrenaline (epinephrine/ norepinephrine)	Acute stress response; affect glucose mobilization and blood flow
Aldosterone	Regulates sodium/potassium balance and blood pressure—can shift with hormone transitions (e.g., PMS, menopause)

Thyroid Gland ***Located in the front of your neck***	
Thyroxine (T4) and triiodothyronine (T3)	Regulate metabolism, energy, temperature, digestion, and influence menstrual regularity, fertility, and ovarian function
Calcitonin	Helps regulate calcium levels (less central to reproductive hormone health, but worth noting)

Placenta ***Located in the upper part of the uterus (during pregnancy)***	
Human chorionic gonadotropin (hCG)	Maintains corpus luteum and progesterone production in early pregnancy
Placental estrogen (mainly Estriol, E3) and progesterone	Support pregnancy, fetal development, and uterine growth
Human placental lactogen (hPL)	Modulates maternal metabolism to support fetal nutrition

Adipose Tissue, Skin, and Peripheral Tissues ***Located all throughout the body***	
Estrone (E1)	Weaker estrogen, mainly produced in fat tissue post-menopause, still influences bones and mood
Leptin	Signals energy availability; influences GnRH and fertility (low levels = disrupted cycles)

Pancreas ***Located in the upper abdomen, behind the stomach***	
Insulin	Enables glucose uptake into cells; supports blood sugar balance, ovulation, and hormone signaling
Glucagon	Opposes insulin; raises blood sugar levels between meals and helps maintain energy homeostasis

Liver ***Located in the upper right abdomen, beneath the diaphragm***	
Sex hormone-binding globulin (SHBG)	Binds estrogen and testosterone; regulates their bioavailability and balance
Thyroxine-binding globulin (TBG)	Transports thyroid hormones (T4 and T3) in the bloodstream; maintains thyroid hormone stability
Insulin-like growth factor-1 (IGF-1)	Mediates growth hormone effects; supports cell growth, metabolism, and ovarian function
Angiotensinogen	Precursor to angiotensin; critical for blood pressure regulation and fluid balance
Hepcidin	Master regulator of iron metabolism; controls absorption and distribution of iron throughout the body

Welcome to the Hormone Group Chat

Your hormones are constantly talking to one another and to various parts of the body. Think of it like a group chat between your brain, your hormone-producing glands (like the thyroid, ovaries, and adrenals), and the organs they send signals to (like the liver, pancreas, and muscles), which can also talk back and carry out functions.

Chemical messages (aka hormones) are sent out, received, and responded to—with new messages sent back in real time based on what's happening. In medicine, we call these *feedback loops*.

For example:

- When estrogen levels rise during your cycle, they send a signal to the hypothalamus and pituitary glands to reduce follicle-stimulating hormone (FSH).
- But right before ovulation, estrogen gets so high it flips the switch and triggers a surge of Luteinizing hormone (LH).

- When stress hormones like cortisol spike up, they suppress reproductive hormone signals.
- If the hormones produced by your thyroid are low, your brain increases thyroid-stimulating hormone (TSH) to stimulate the thyroid to produce more—until the levels are back in balance.

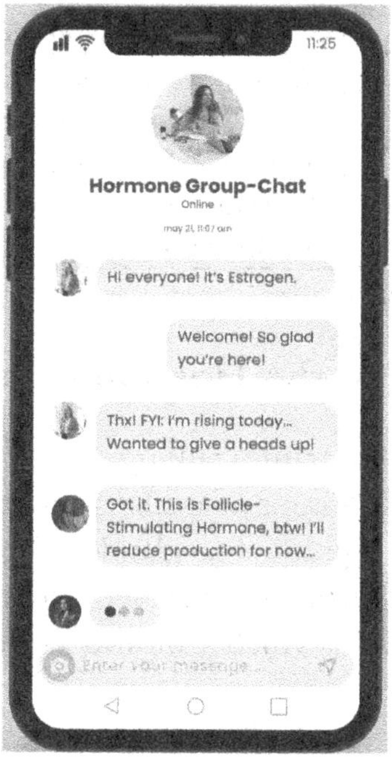
11:25
Hormone Group-Chat
Online
Hi everyone! It's Estrogen.
Welcome! So glad you're here!
Thx! FYI: I'm rising today... Wanted to give a heads up!
Got it. This is Follicle-Stimulating Hormone, btw! I'll reduce production for now...

Every moment of your life, there's an invisible conversation happening inside your body.

This is your body's internal feedback loops, or checks-and-balances system. It keeps your hormones within just the right range—not too much, not too little, just right—based on what's needed in the moment. Or at least, that's what is *supposed* to happen. Sometimes, the group chat goes haywire.

Often, by the time a woman comes into my clinic, the communication breakdown has been happening for a long time. Years. Maybe decades.

Optimal communication can be restored, but it takes time. The following section explains what this looked like for one client, Helene.

Our Bodies Keep Score

Helene was 43 when she came to see me. She was experiencing textbook perimenopausal shifts: hot flashes, night sweats, hair loss, low libido, feeling blue and anxious, weight gain, and heavy bleeding.

Her labs told a fuller story: early-stage type 2 diabetes, iron-deficiency anemia, and late-stage perimenopause (happening earlier than most). A mammogram revealed a suspicious mass. An ultrasound showed a 7 cm uterine fibroid. Her doctor had put her on birth control in her teens to regulate her cycle, and she stayed on it until her early 30s, when she stopped to conceive in her mid-30s. After childbirth, no one revisited her hormone health again, even though the same irregular periods returned.

On paper, Helene looked like she had been doing all the right things. She ate balanced meals and exercised consistently. But she had a love of wine, sugary snacks, and treats, and carried the chronic stress of a high-profile job. Like many women, her thinking was, "If I'm still able to work and carry out my daily responsibilities, if I'm not in a full-blown crisis, then everything is fine."

But everything was not fine. And Helene noticed that she felt increasingly worse. She thought hormone replacement therapy (HRT), also known as menopausal hormone therapy (MHT), might be her magic fix, the thing that would finally make everything click back into place. But by the time she came to me, she was already living with metabolic syndrome, elevated cancer risk, and likely irreversible hair loss. It didn't happen overnight. It was decades in the making. The hormonal highways in her body had been disrupted for a long time, and now, in her 40s, she was *really* feeling it.

Undoing is harder than prevention. And our bodies keep score.

Running tests on Helene helped us pinpoint what was out of whack, so we could develop a wellness plan to bring her back into balance. By carrying out the plan and testing several times over many months, we could see her hormone levels change and return to optimal ranges. This provided proof that the plan was working, and Helene could see and feel the difference. She had a feeling of internal control and motivation to keep going.

When Women Understand How Their Bodies Work, They Can Become Leaders Rather Than Passive Participants in Their Lives

If you are reading this book later in life, know that it is never too late to get educated about your hormones: the sacred messengers of the body.

It is never too late to nudge the nose of the airplane a few degrees to the right or left and get your life moving in the direction you want.

It is never too late to create optimal health.

As the proverb goes, "The best time to plant a tree was 10 years ago. The second best time is now."

In your 30s, 40s, and 50s, you still have a great deal of life ahead of you. The years ahead should feel incredible, not painful, and not just tolerable. Your time is now.

Key Takeaways

- Hormones are messengers—chemical signals that travel through your bloodstream and lymph fluid, delivering instructions to keep everything in your body running smoothly.
- Your body produces more than 50 hormones. Each one performs important tasks in your body. Estrogen, progesterone, testosterone, cortisol, and melatonin are the top five to remember. T3 and T4 (both produced by your thyroid) are two other hormones that every woman should know.

- There's constant communication happening between your brain, your hormone-producing glands, and the organs they signal, which also respond—creating a feedback loop.
- Sometimes, due to stress, nutrient deficiencies, and other factors, communication channels can be disrupted.
- When hormone levels are too high or too low or when there's a communication breakdown, this leads to uncomfortable symptoms. Symptoms are your body's way of saying, "Something is off. Please help!"
- Although hormones affect everything from metabolism to bone density to sleep cycles and beyond, they are deeply misunderstood, even by many medical professionals.
- Closing the knowledge gap will take time. When women (like you) get educated about their own bodies, this accelerates progress. Change starts with *you.*

Notes

1. "Closing the Women's Health Gap: A $1 Trillion Opportnity to Improve Lives and Economies." World Economic Forum. 2024. https://www.weforum.org/publications/closing-the-women-s-health-gap-a-1-trillion-opportunity-to-improve-lives-and-economies/.
2. "Closing the Women's Health Gap: A $1 Trillion Opportunity to Improve Lives and Economies." McKinsey Health Institute. World Economic Forum. 2024. https://www.weforum.org/publications/closing-the-women-s-health-gap-a-1-trillion-opportunity-to-improve-lives-and-economies/.
3. Dusenbery, M. *Doing harm: The truth about how bad medicine and lazy science leave women dismissed, misdiagnosed, and sick.* HarperCollins, 2018.

4. "What Is the Gender Health Gap?". *Evvy*. Cassano, Olivia. Updated 29 December 2025. Available from: https://www.evvy.com/blog/gender-health-gap.
5. "S.1 - 103rd Congress (1993-1994): National Institutes of Health Revitalization Act of 1993." *Congress.gov.* Library of Congress. 10 June 1993, https://www.congress.gov/bill/103rd-congress/senate-bill/1.

Chapter 2

Endocrine Evolution: Hormones and the Stages of a Woman's Life

I'll never forget her.

Amelia was 40 when she first came to see me—exhausted, discouraged, and caught in a cycle of chronic sinus and respiratory infections that wouldn't let up. She had two young kids and caught everything they brought home, but unlike her family, who bounced back in days, Amelia was left wiped out for weeks or months at a time. Round after round of antibiotics only made things worse; gut disruption, fatigue, low mood, brain fog, and anxiety. Her body was crying out, and perimenopause was right around the corner.

Her immunologist had finally diagnosed her with low immunoglobulin levels and reluctantly prescribed her subcutaneous immunoglobulin replacement therapy. It was a hopeful step but still just palliative, and not necessarily a root-cause resolution. It was costly as a therapy she'd have to take for the rest of her life, and so she hadn't yet started it when she came to me. I was her last resort and outside-the-box approach. Every specialist she'd seen over the past decade—primary care, pulmonology, gastroenterology, immunology—had worked her up for everything from rare infections to autoimmune disease to cancer and genetics. And yet, no one could explain *why* her immune system was flailing.

At first glance, she was the picture of wellness. Athletic, lean, glowing skin, clean organic diet. She didn't drink, didn't smoke, took good quality supplements, and ran several miles a day. She practiced yoga regularly, clocked seven to eight hours of sleep per night, and had never been on prescription medication. On paper and to the outside world—Amelia was "healthy."

But when I sat with her, heard her full story, and looked at her labs, I saw something deeper. Her body was working *so hard* to maintain a standard of health that, underneath, wasn't sustainable.

When I reviewed her labs, the only abnormality noted was a low IgG level—her immunoglobulin antibody levels. But more shocking than what *was* tested was what *wasn't*. Despite over a decade of declining resilience, no one had ever run a comprehensive hormone panel. Not even once. Aside from an annual thyroid-stimulating hormone (TSH) blood test, her hormonal story had been completely ignored. Absent.

So, I asked about her cycles.

That's when the real story came into view.

Decades of Dysregulation

In her 20s and 30s, Amelia had long periods of time, sometimes months, without a period. Sometimes she didn't ovulate at all. Her OB/GYN wasn't concerned, chalking it up to stress and telling her, "It's nothing to worry about unless you miss more than three months in a row." Since she had conceived easily and carried both pregnancies without issue, no red flags were ever raised by her or her doctors.

But I saw it clearly: Amelia had likely been hormonally suppressed (hypoestrogenic) for decades, verging on hypothalamic amenorrhea, a condition where physical body stress can impact signals from the brain that lead to more hormone suppression body-wide. The longer we talked, the more I suspected a classic case of relative energy deficiency in sport (RED-S), a condition initially identified in female athletes that was formerly termed the *Female Athlete Triad*: overexercise (or *overstress*), under-fueling, and menstrual dysfunction. It was one of the most overlooked root causes of hormone imbalance in high-functioning women.

Amelia's relentless drive to achieve—in fitness, at work, at home, in all aspects of life—was taking a toll on her body, because she wasn't resting and refueling enough to keep up with the demands she placed upon herself, extracting too much, without sufficient replenishment. Amelia is what I call an Achiever, one of the three Hormone Types that you'll meet in Part Two. For many Achievers, like Amelia, there's a tendency to push to the brink of exhaustion, which begins early in life and carries onward, leading to bigger and bigger consequences over time.

And so, we tested the hormone labs that were missing. Not just for fertility, but to understand her complete endocrine picture: her ovarian reserve, adrenal resilience, and neurohormonal signaling.

I ran the following lab tests for Amelia:

- Estradiol, follicle-stimulating hormone (FSH), luteinizing hormone (LH) (Days 2–5) (shows if you are nearing perimenopause or not)
- Anti-Müllerian hormone (AMH) (gives a picture of ovarian reserve and reproductive stage)
- Progesterone (Days 18–24) (tells us if you are ovulating)
- Free and total testosterone (shows if you are low in testosterone or have signs of excess/androgen dominance)
- DHEA-S (shows how active your adrenal glands are)

- Prolactin (shows if your pituitary gland is affecting menstrual cycles or if there is a mass growing that could be impacting your cycles)
- Fasting serum cortisol and a four-point salivary cortisol rhythm (shows stress rhythms across the day)
- Full thyroid panel with antibodies (can influence periods and much more)

The results told the story her body had been trying to share for years: she was hormonally depleted—and not just estrogen but across the board. Her endocrine system was underpowered, and her immune system was paying the price.

Nobody had ever suggested that her immune issues could be *hormonal*. Not even the top specialists in Los Angeles.

Her distress wasn't just about the ovaries. It was about the entire endocrine system, the hypothalamus, pituitary, adrenals, thyroid, and ovaries, all of which had been dysregulated for years.

As we discussed briefly in the previous chapter, the 50+ hormones in a woman's body are continually talking to one another, like a group chat between the hormones, hormone-producing glands, and the organs that receive and send back signals. Many of these communication patterns are set during puberty and continue for decades. When one part of the system is under pressure, the entire network feels the strain. The ovaries are often the last to speak up, but by then, the conversation has already been strained for years.

Traffic Jams on the Hormonal Highways

Imagine driving a car down a clear, open freeway. No traffic jams. No obstructions. No delays. When your hormone highways are functioning optimally, that's what it's like. Smooth, flowing communication. However, just like a freeway can get jammed up, this can happen in your body too. Chronically elevated stress levels, inflammation, nutrient deficiencies, emotional and physical trauma, and many other factors can disrupt the flow of communication between your brain, glands, and organs. The result? Roadblocks and traffic jams.

What happens when hormonal communication channels get disrupted? You don't feel well. You start noticing symptoms, signaling that something is not right. Over time, if unattended, you may develop a serious condition.

In the state of Maine, where I live, the I-95 interstate freeway intersects with the 295, and the 202, and many other highways and roads. All the hormonal communication highways in your body are interconnected, too. When one is disrupted, the others can get thrown out of sync as well.

That's why stress affects ovulation.

That's why insulin resistance affects testosterone and estrogen.

That's why thyroid issues can mimic menopause or premenstrual syndrome (PMS).

That's why synthetic birth control shuts down the whole ovulatory feedback loop, thereby inhibiting pregnancy.

When a woman visits my clinic, she often wants to know, **"Are my hormone levels too high, too low, or in the right zone?"** This is a great question—but it's not the *only* question.

While levels do matter, what's equally important is asking, **"Are the communication channels working properly?"** Is there a roadblock somewhere in the body that's interfering with communication between the brain, glands, and organs? If so, how can we restore communication and get the highway working properly again?

To achieve optimal health, it usually takes more than a pill or injection to adjust hormone levels—although this may be part of the treatment plan. But it's also about improving communication throughout the entire system. It's truly a whole-systems and whole-body approach.

Many women experience hormonal communication pathway disruption at some point in their lives. This is why one woman might reach menopause at 35 and another at 55 and why their symptoms can look completely different. It's why some women develop osteopenia or osteoporosis in their 40s, while others never do. Why some face the worst depression and anxiety of their lives in perimenopause, while others glide through it. Why some experience sudden weight gain, metabolic chaos, immune issues, or gut dysfunction for years *before* they ever miss a period.

The longer we go without understanding what's really going on, the more years are lost not feeling our best. And the harder it can hit when menopause arrives.

Bonus Chapter

Your body has eight major hormonal communication highways, known as axes. Two of the most important axes? The hypothalamic-pituitary-thyroid-adrenal-ovarian (HPTAO) axis and the gut-brain-hormone axis (also called the microbiota-gut-brain axis).

For a deep dive into these axes, how they can get jammed up, and how to restore optimal functioning, I wrote a **bonus chapter**. Scan the code to read it.

If you're a healthcare provider or anyone who wants to learn more about these communication pathways, check it out.

Hormones Influence Everything

Amelia is the perfect example of a woman whose health issues got misdiagnosed and misunderstood—because her symptoms didn't look "hormonal." In our society, when someone says, "My hormone levels are out of whack," most people picture a woman with terrible PMS, mood swings, or hot flashes. You know, "hormonal stuff." They don't picture a woman with an underfunctioning immune system who keeps getting sick.

This is one of the main reasons why I felt called to write this book: to educate women about the fact that hormones impact *every* system in your body, not just reproduction and your menstrual cycle. Your nervous system, digestive system, respiratory system, every system, including (as in Amelia's case) the immune system, are all impacted when certain hormones are not in the optimal ranges.

Amelia's suppressed immune system was the canary in the coal mine. Her sinus infections, low resilience, and fatigue just the tip of the iceberg.

Hers may be a more extreme presentation, but this pattern is not rare. Crippling anxiety, brain fog, and depression in our teens, 20s, and 30s. Sudden weight gain. Inexplicable sleepless nights. A disappearing libido. These aren't just mood or motivation problems. They're often hormonal. And women are told, "There's nothing we can do about this right now. Wait until menopause, and then we can put you on an HRT prescription." But "waiting until menopause" isn't an effective strategy. It leads to years of needless suffering. And while she is "waiting," the negative snowball of hormonal dysregulation often gets worse.

I'll admit, I see everything through the lens of hormones, but here's the truth: estrogen is immunoprotective. It plays a vital role in maintaining mucosal barriers, including in the lungs and sinuses. Without enough estrogen, these tissues become more vulnerable to infection, inflammation, and immune dysregulation.

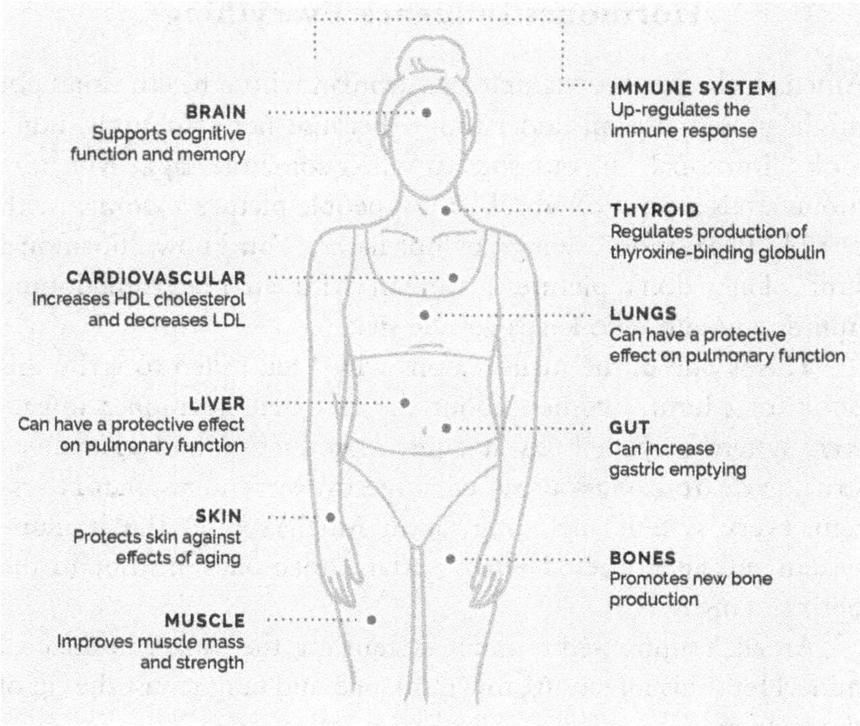

Figure 2.1 The role of estrogen in the body.

Progesterone is also powerfully protective—especially in calming inflammation and regulating immune responses. It acts as a natural immunomodulator, helping prevent immune overreactions while supporting mucosal healing and repair. When it's low, women are more prone to anxiety, sleep disruption, and systemic inflammation—all of which further weaken immune resilience. See Figure 2.1.

And it's not just estrogen and progesterone. The other key players in the HPTAO axis, such as thyroid hormones and cortisol, can, if dysregulated, impact immune function. Chronically high cortisol can alter inflammation pathways and weaken the body's ability to repair. Suboptimal thyroid function impairs cellular metabolic and immune function. When this intricate hormonal symphony falls out of tune, the immune system bears the brunt—leaving women like Amelia more vulnerable to infections, fatigue, and slower recovery, even when everything "looks fine" on paper without a closer hormonal look.

Amelia's immune system didn't fail out of nowhere. Her story started unraveling in her 20s, when her hormonal resilience was already slipping. It just took two decades—and one doctor willing to look deeper—for someone to see the whole picture.

Your Body's Endocrine Evolution

Throughout your life, your endocrine system—the intricate messenger network that governs your hormones—is in constant motion. It doesn't just "turn on" at puberty and "turn off" at menopause. It evolves. It adapts. It responds to your environment, your stress levels, your sleep, your nutrition, your relationships, and even your thoughts. It is beautifully dynamic, never static.

While your endocrine system is continually evolving, there are a few critical moments in your lifetime when the changes are especially dramatic and happen in an accelerated manner—such as puberty, pregnancy, postpartum, and menopause, to name a few.

During these transitional moments, a woman is more vulnerable. Many complex processes are happening in her body. She can become hormonally dysregulated more easily. The actions you take during these critical moments set the stage for either a positive snowball effect or a negative one in the years ahead.

Let's look at some of the major moments in a woman's endocrine evolution. . .

An Endocrine Timeline: A Woman's Hormonal Life over the Years

In Utero (Before Birth)

By 20 weeks of gestation, a female fetus carries about six to seven million eggs (oocytes). By birth, less than one million remain, and by puberty, less than 300,000. Of these, only about 400–500 will ever be ovulated across a lifetime. This ovarian supply is not just

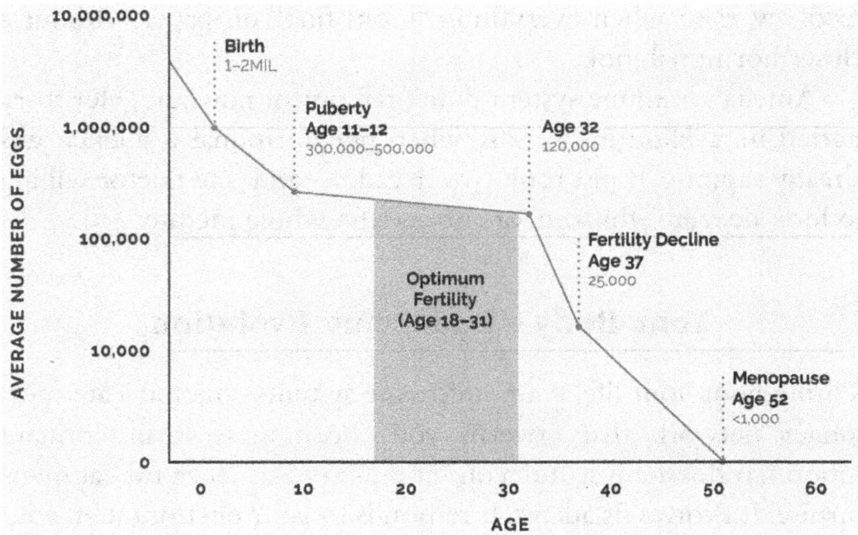

Figure 2.2 The production of eggs over an average human lifetime.

about fertility; it sets the stage for hormonal resilience throughout life. The health of those eggs and the rhythms they govern determine bone density, brain health, cardiovascular strength, long-term metabolic stability, and more. See Figure 2.2.

Infancy and Early Childhood

Even as a very young child, hormonal patterns begin shaping health right away. Melatonin production in the pineal gland ramps up in infancy, establishing circadian rhythms that regulate sleep, brain development, and, later, reproductive cycles. Healthy sleep in childhood programs the hypothalamic-pituitary-thyroid-adrenal-ovarian (HPTAO) axis for a lifetime of hormonal health.

This is why a healthy lifestyle—good sleep habits, whole foods and minimal processed junk, time outdoors, physical activity, loving connections with parents and other caregivers—is so critical for children. Patterns are being established now that build momentum in the years ahead, creating either a positive snowball effect or a negative one. See Figure 2.3.

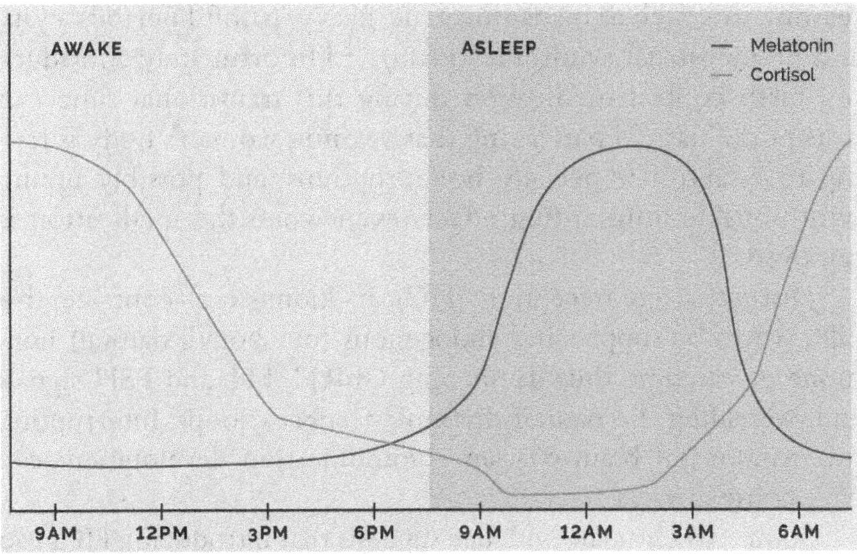

Figure 2.3 The production of cortisol and melatonin throughout the day.

Puberty (Typically 8–13 Years)

A surge of estrogen and progesterone activates breast development, menstruation, and the growth of secondary sexual characteristics. Testosterone—often overlooked in girls—also rises, fueling confidence, strength, and motivation. The hormonal symphony here isn't just about reproduction; it's about brain wiring, bone building, and metabolic set points that can influence health for decades.

An important note regarding puberty and birth control: puberty is a time of great transition, and similarly to perimenopause, it can bring with it irregular ovulation and irregular bleeding patterns. On average, girls can take three to four years after menarche (the first menstrual period) until they reach a predictable and regular bleeding cycle.

This transitional time of irregularity is normal; however, girls are sometimes offered birth control pills to "jumpstart" or "regulate" their cycles—as though something is wrong that needs to be fixed. Some girls are offered the pill at a young age for other reasons, too, such as managing acne, heavy/painful periods, cysts, and premenstrual syndrome (PMS).[1,2] Unfortunately, introducing birth control medication during this transitional time can disrupt the natural patterning that a young woman's body is trying to establish (especially bone, rhythms, and possibly brain), with possible long-lasting effects even when the medication is removed.[3,4]

Hormonal contraception (HC), including oral contraceptive pills, works by suppressing endogenous (our body's natural) hormone production, thus dampening GnRH, LH, and FSH signals and overriding the natural rhythmic feedback loops. Interrupting this window of brain-ovarian communication development can have consequences.

Some early human evidence suggests that introducing HCs too early may alter HPA axis (stress system) responses, brain function, and stress reactivity. Limited data suggests that adolescent HC users as a group show higher rate of antidepressant use and suicidal behavior in some cohorts.[5]

As the American Psychological Association reports, "One troubling finding: taking hormonal contraceptives during adolescence is linked to a higher risk of developing major depressive disorder in adulthood."[6] The APA cites the work of Frances Chen, PhD, a professor of psychology who studies how hormones influence social and emotional health. Chen and her colleagues conducted a research project that tracked data from teenage girls (ages 13–15) before they began taking the pill and for years afterward. Their findings, as the APA states, "suggests there may be a long-term effect of these synthetic hormones on the way the brain develops during adolescence."

This makes sense, as puberty is a critical window for the HPG axis to develop its communication pathways. The HPG axis governs the hormonal interplay between the brain and the ovaries, orchestrating ovulation and cyclical hormone rhythms—a foundational system that is fine-tuned during this stage. Disrupting this patterning can have unintended consequences that we are only just now beginning to understand.[7] The gradual post-menarche settling of regular cyclicity isn't arbitrary: it reflects the brain-ovary communication (HPG axis) and brain-stress communication (HPA axis) evolving into a whole-body health support system for life.

The Reproductive Years (Typically 13–35 Years)

Across monthly cycles, the very important hormones (VIHs, which you might recall from Chapter 1) play starring roles:

- **Estrogen** sharpens memory, boosts mood, and protects cardiovascular health.
- **Progesterone** calms the mind, supports sleep, and balances estrogen's growth-promoting effects.
- **Testosterone** powers libido, muscle mass, and drive.
- **Cortisol** fine-tunes energy and stress resilience.
- **Melatonin** ensures rest and rhythm.
- **Thyroid hormones (T3 and T4)** set the metabolic tempo.

The balance of these hormones protects against early heart disease, osteoporosis, autoimmune conditions, and mood disorders.

Remember back in Chapter 1 when I shared how many medical students struggle to map out a menstrual cycle and the hormones involved? They'd never been taught this information. Maybe you never received this lesson, either. Let's change that, right now.

Take a good look at these graphs—study them and then try sketching them out yourself on a blank sheet of paper (yes, really. . . and no peeking). I promise, this exercise will lock the cycle into your memory and give you a powerful tool for understanding your own body. See Figure 2.4.

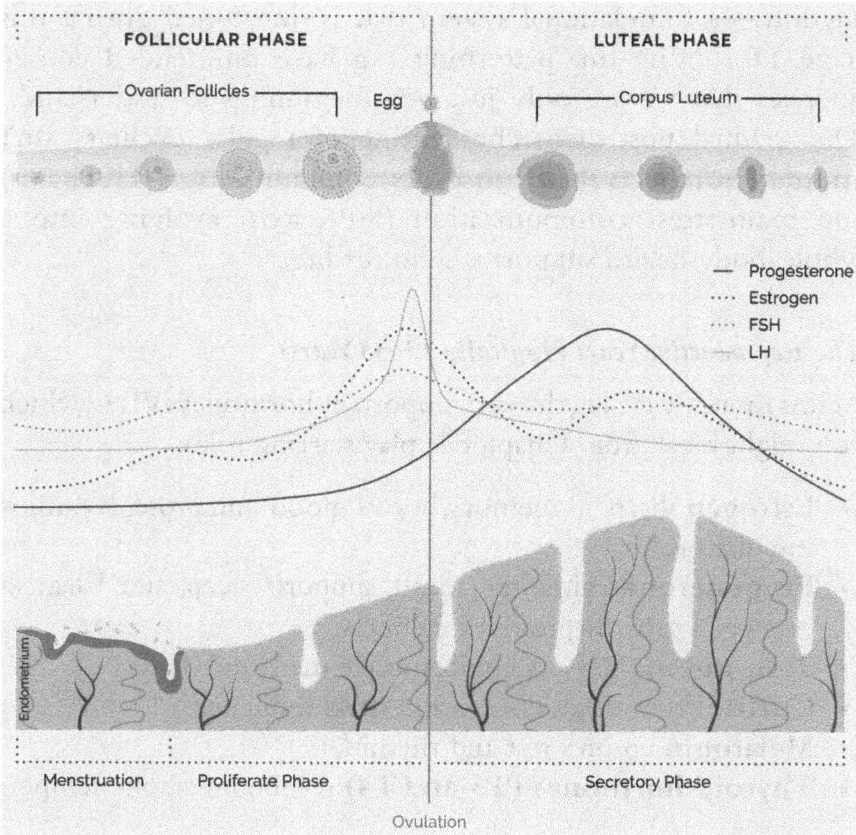

Figure 2.4 The human menstrual cycle.

Here is a summary of what's happening throughout a typical menstrual cycle during the reproductive years.

The Four Phases of the Menstrual Cycle

- *Menstrual phase:* Shedding of the uterine lining. Hormone levels are at their lowest
- *Follicular phase:* Follicles in the ovary grow, and estrogen begins rebuilding the uterine lining
- *Ovulatory phase:* A surge of hormones triggers ovulation (egg release)
- *Luteal phase:* Progesterone stabilizes and enriches the uterine lining in case of implantation

Key Hormones and Their Roles

- **FSH:** Stimulates ovarian follicles to grow and mature an egg
- **LH:** Surges mid-cycle to trigger ovulation
- **Estrogen:** Builds and thickens the uterine lining and also primes cervical mucus for sperm entry
- **Progesterone:** Protects and stabilizes the uterine lining after ovulation, preparing it for potential implantation

Impact on the Uterine Lining

- During the *menstrual phase*, the lining is shed due to low estrogen and progesterone.
- In the *follicular phase*, rising estrogen rebuilds and thickens the lining.
- At *ovulation*, estrogen peaks, and the lining becomes fertile and receptive.
- In the *luteal phase*, progesterone (with support from estrogen) stabilizes and enriches the lining. If pregnancy doesn't occur, progesterone drops, and the lining is released, starting the next period.

Menstrual Cycle Hormone Recap

- FSH = Follicle starter (grows the eggs)
- LH = Ovulation trigger (releases the eggs)
- Estrogen = Builder (thickens the uterine lining)
- Progesterone = Protector (stabilizes the lining)

Think of it like gardening: FSH plants the seed, estrogen grows the garden, LH releases the flower, and progesterone tends and protects it—until it's either harvested (pregnancy) or cleared for a fresh start (menstruation).

Pregnancy and Postpartum

During pregnancy, estrogen and progesterone soar to levels 10–100× higher than at any other time, shaping mood, immunity, and even the brain. Postpartum, these hormones steeply decline, combined with sleep-disrupting drops in melatonin and surges of cortisol.

These rapid and drastic hormonal changes coincide with a massive identity shift—the transition from woman to mother and everything this entails. Round-the-clock caregiving responsibilities. Excitement about this new season of life. Grief for the old life that no longer exists. Pressure (whether societally imposed, self-imposed, or both) to perform at a high level and be the best possible mother. All while recovering from the demands of pregnancy and birth. All of this, alongside the big chemical swings, make this one of the most hormonally vulnerable times in a woman's life.

Vulnerable postpartum women—the ones who are suffering intensely and who are the most at-risk for conditions that can escalate to a serious or even life-threatening level—often struggle to get the care they need. They are too overwhelmed to seek help (trying to log into your health insurance website to search for providers in your network is extremely difficult when you have a newborn shrieking in your ear or when you are too sleep-deprived to think straight) or hope that at some point, things will just "get better" on their own. But unfortunately, for many, the negative snowball doesn't just vanish—it continues to build speed and force.

As the World Health Organization reports, "More than a third of women experience lasting health problems after childbirth," citing a study that shows "a high burden of postnatal conditions that persist in the months or even years after giving birth."[8] Pain during intercourse, anxiety, depression, and many other conditions continue, or worsen, when postpartum women don't have the support they need to thrive. See Figure 2.5.

Perimenopause (Typically 35–50 Years)

Egg supply declines more rapidly: from less than 25,000 at age 37 to fewer than 1,000 at menopause. Estrogen and progesterone

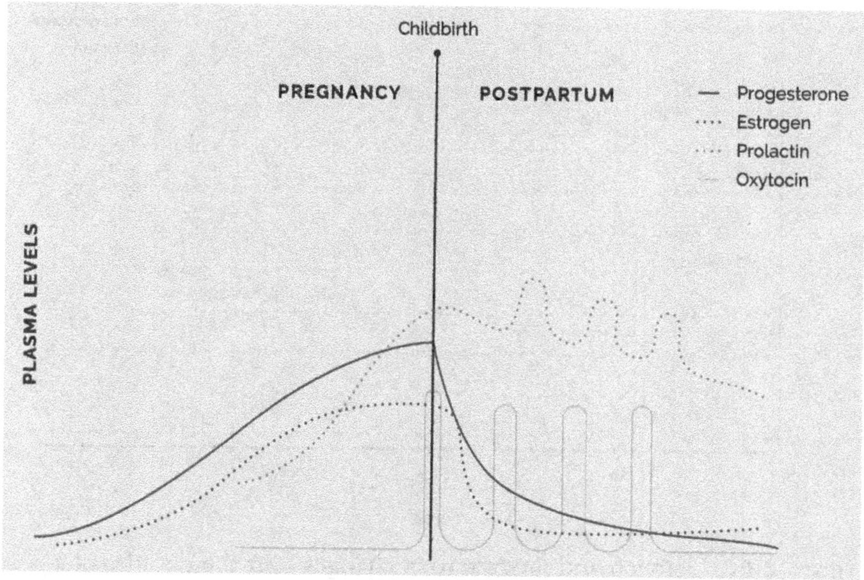

Figure 2.5 Hormonal changes during and after pregnancy.

begin to fluctuate wildly, creating symptoms like heavy or irregular periods, sleep disruption, anxiety, brain fog, and weight changes. Cortisol often rises in compensation, straining your body's resilience.

This is the critical window where proactive hormone care—including stress management tools, deep restorative sleep, movement, nutrition, targeted supplements, a strong support network, and in some instances, bio-identical hormone replacement therapy—pays off. Support here changes the trajectory of how women age. When patients come to me during this window of time, we can make powerful changes that can alter the second half of a woman's life. See Figure 2.6.

Menopause and Beyond (Typically 50+)

Once the ovarian egg reserve is depleted, estrogen and progesterone production plummet. Without proactive hormone care strategies, risks for osteoporosis, dementia, cardiovascular disease, and

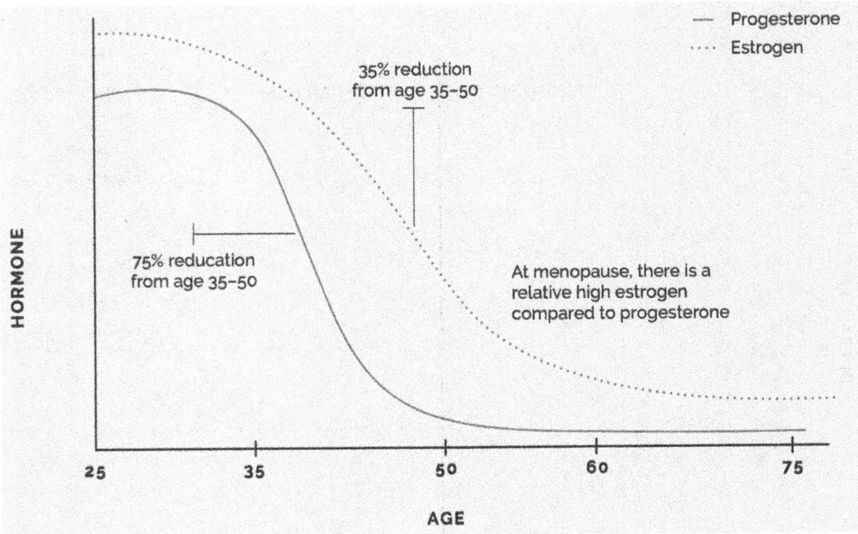

Figure 2.6 Estrogen and progesterone changes over the decades of a woman's life.

metabolic dysfunction rise sharply. Testosterone, thyroid hormones (T3 and T4), cortisol, and melatonin still matter deeply—though at lower levels, they can still be optimized for vitality, strength, and longevity.

Ideal Versus Dysregulated Endocrine Evolution

Starting when you are a fetus in your mother's womb, all the way to puberty, then moving along to pregnancy (if you choose to have children), then eventually perimenopause, menopause, and beyond, your endocrine system continues to evolve and change. This is normal and natural. It's what is supposed to happen. It's the journey of life. However, there is a big difference between ideal evolution and *dysregulated* evolution.

In an ideal scenario, your hormonal shifts follow a graceful progression, like a symphony playing in rhythm with your life stages. These shifts are biologically designed to support your energy, immunity, metabolism, mood, cognition, and reproductive function. With the proper support, they can be seamless. You're meant to ebb and flow—not crash and burn.

But when the endocrine system is disrupted—whether by chronic stress, poor sleep, environmental toxins, blood sugar instability, medications, illnesses, or simply being dismissed by doctors who say "your labs look fine"—those changes no longer feel graceful. They feel chaotic. You lose your rhythm. You lose your sense of self. Some body systems may start to show signs of imbalance.

This dysregulation doesn't happen overnight. It accumulates. It snowballs over time—until one day, you're sitting across from a doctor being handed birth control or antidepressants, wondering how things got so far off track.

The good news? Your endocrine system is designed for restoration. You can course-correct. You can realign with your body's natural intelligence. And the earlier you start, especially in your teens, 20s, 30s, and early 40s, the more powerful your results.

Hormone Powered exists to help you do precisely that: to decode what your hormones are telling you and to guide you toward that *ideal* progression—one that leads to vitality, resilience, and radiance through every stage of life.

Getting the Endocrine System Back on Track

When Amelia, the patient I mentioned at the top of this chapter, came into my clinic at age 40 suffering from chronic illnesses and feeling truly miserable, her endocrine system had been dysregulated for many years. My job was to help get her endocrine system back on track, back to the ideal evolution we want a woman to experience.

If I had seen Amelia a couple of decades earlier, back when she was in her 20s or early 30s, my treatment approach would have been different. I likely would have started with what I consider foundational and first-line, focusing on restoring her natural hormonal rhythms and cyclicity through lifestyle changes, nutrition, botanicals, and targeted supplements.

But by age 40, Amelia was a woman with *years* of suboptimal hormone exposure—a body deprived of its natural hormonal protection and labs showing a low remaining egg reserve, which meant a low remaining ability to produce her protective amount of estrogen and progesterone. Because of her age and the severity of her situation, I felt she needed a more integrative approach. Bringing the best of both worlds—pharmaceutical and naturopathic—together. When the gap between how you currently feel and how you want to feel is *very* wide, sometimes you need a more assertive approach to close it.

Amelia had never been interested in synthetic birth control, and (aside from the antibiotics she'd been put on to manage her chronic infections) she tended to veer away from prescription medications. She preferred natural supplements and homeopathic remedies when possible. But once I explained the concept of bio-identical hormone replacement therapy (BHRT) and how estrogen and progesterone impact immunity—not just fertility—she was open and curious.

Together, we chose a both/and strategy:

- A body-protective level of bio-identical estradiol (a type of estrogen), plus progesterone to balance and support, not enough to entirely suppress her own body's endogenous hormone production, but to lift her baseline
- Nutritional repair with micronutrient repletion and a reverse dieting protocol (a gradual process of increasing caloric intake after a period of food restriction, to boost the metabolism) to support her adrenal and thyroid health
- Nervous system support to downshift out of sympathetic overdrive (her body has been stuck in "fight or flight" mode for too long, and Amelia needed to retrain her body to learn how to settle, relax, and experience safety once again)

- Botanicals to support the top-down hormone signaling: brain health, HPA-axis regulation, and circadian alignment
- A rhythm of care that overall felt doable and sustainable with the big, busy life she was living

Although BHRT was part of Amelia's overall wellness plan, it was just one of many components. Hormone replacement therapy, alone, is never a complete solution. Because Amelia was willing to make changes in multiple areas, her body responded beautifully.

Within just the first month, she messaged me this:

> "I'm trying not to jinx it, but I've officially been on the plan we've put together for the past 30 days, and I've never felt better. Every day, the color of my snot and lung congestion has gotten lighter and lighter. Yesterday I felt like a normal human. I didn't need to start antibiotics because I no longer feel sick. Today I neti-potted and—nothing. Just water. That hasn't happened in a year. I am in shock. Also, I realized I wasn't cold for the first time in forever—my internal body temp finally feels right. I'm warm and cozy and comfortable again. . .I'm kinda freaking out—in a good way."

This is what happens when we stop separating the systems of the body. When we start asking why, not just what. When we look beyond symptoms to one of the most foundational networking systems that touches nearly every tissue in the body, our endocrine system and the hormones that it produces. And, when we trust women's stories and connect the dots that others miss.

Your endocrine system is designed to evolve through the seasons of your life, but this evolution doesn't have to feel painful, and if it is, that's a sign that something is out of balance. I wish I had a time machine and could have supported Amelia in her teens, 20s, and 30s, preventing years of poor health that eroded her quality of life. However, even in your 40s and 50s, it is not too late to restore your endocrine system. When you are older, as many of my patients are, it often requires "more" (more support, more time, more patience, sometimes, introducing bioidentical hormones and other modalities) to get the endocrine system back on track if it has been derailed for decades, but it is doable.

Wherever you are on the endocrine evolution timeline, there is hope, and there is a path forward for you.

Key Takeaways

Hormones in your body impact everything, not just your menstrual cycle, fertility, and reproduction.

- Your nervous system, digestive system, respiratory system, immune system, and other systems are all impacted when certain hormones are too low or too high.
- Throughout your life, your endocrine system—the system that produces and regulates hormones—is continually changing and evolving.
- Endocrine evolution is normal. However, there is a big difference between an ideal evolution versus a dysregulated evolution.
- For many women, due to chronic stress, nutritional deficiencies, the unintended consequences of certain medications, and more, the endocrine system's natural evolution gets thrown off course.
- The signs of dysregulated endocrine evolution start out small but often grow bigger and more severe over time.

- There are several key transitions in a woman's life when her hormonal landscape undergoes especially big changes: in utero, early childhood, puberty, pregnancy, postpartum, perimenopause, and menopause.
- During these transitions, a woman's endocrine system is especially vulnerable. However, these transitions also provide a window of opportunity to be proactive about hormonal care, make positive changes, and lay the groundwork for optimal health.
- Even if your endocrine evolution has been off-track for years, or even decades, you can get things back on track. The earlier you address the issues, the better—but it is never too late.

Notes

1. Bonny, A., et al. (2015). Hormonal Contraceptive Agents: A Need for Pediatric-Specific Studies. *Pediatrics*, 135, 4–6. https://doi.org/10.1542/peds.2014-1511.
2. Van Hooff, M., et al. (1998). The Use of Oral Contraception by Adolescents for Contraception, Menstrual Cycle Problems or Acne. *Acta Obstetricia et Gynecologica Scandinavica*, 77. https://doi.org/10.1034/j.1600-0412.1998.770905.x.
3. Zettermark, S., et al. (2018). Hormonal Contraception Increases the Risk of Psychotropic Drug Use in Adolescent Girls but Not in Adults: A Pharmacoepidemiological Study on 800 000 Swedish Women. *PLOS ONE*, 13. https://doi.org/10.1371/journal.pone.0194773.
4. Daya, M., et al. (2022). P07 Hormonal Contraceptives: Safe for Use in Adolescent Girls? *Archives of Disease in Childhood*, 107, e25. https://doi.org/10.1136/archdischild-2022-nppg.16.

5. Skovlund, C., et al. (2017). Association of Hormonal Contraception with Suicide Attempts and Suicides. *The American Journal of Psychiatry*, 175, 4, 336–342. https://doi.org/10.1176/appi.ajp.2017.17060616.
6. "How Birth Control Pills Affect the Brain." American Psychological Association. Z. Abrams. 2025. https://www.apa.org/monitor/2025/04-05/birth-control-brain.
7. Høgsted, E. S., et al. (2021). Stress-Hormone Dynamics and Working Memory in Healthy Women Who Use Oral Contraceptives Versus Non-Users. *Frontiers in Endocrinology*. https://www.frontiersin.org/journals/endocrinology/articles/10.3389/fendo.2021.731994/full.
8. "More Than a Third of Women Experience Lasting Health Problems After Childbirth, New Research Shows." World Health Organization. WHO. 2023. https://www.who.int/news/item/07-12-2023-more-than-a-third-of-women-experience-lasting-health-problems-after-childbirth.

Part Two

FIND OUT YOUR TYPE

After passing my board examination to become a licensed naturopathic physician, I did a postdoctoral research fellowship in the field of women's health, which led to being published in several peer-reviewed medical journals. Although I am no longer a full-time researcher and now run a women's health clinic, I still bring this research-focused perspective into my work today. I aim to be as evidence informed as possible and to serve as a bridge between conventional and naturopathic medicine. I'm the kind of doctor who often says to a patient, "You should trust your intuition, absolutely. Intuition is powerful. And, let's confirm that your intuition is correct by doing lab testing."

Because of my research background, I have been trained to analyze large amounts of data and hunt for patterns. Throughout my career, treating thousands of women, I have noticed three patterns that emerge consistently. I call these Hormone Types.

What Are Hormone Types?

When it comes to their hormonal health, most women fall into one of three categories, which I refer to as Hormone Types. The three main Hormone Types are:

The Caretaker	The Achiever	The Survivor

In the next three chapters, you will:

- Meet each type and learn her strengths, challenges, and needs
- Learn what's happening from a biomedical perspective, including the hormonal dysregulation that is most common for each type
- Begin seeing how you can tweak your wellness plan based on your type

To define these three types, I drew from my naturopathic training, my specialized training in the endocrine system, hormone production, and regulation, my medical research background, and my studies in ancient traditions such as Ayurvedic doshas. All of these, combined with my experiences working with thousands of patients, hearing their symptoms and their stories, running their lab tests, and analyzing the results, are what clarified these three types.

How to Find Out Your Type

My team and I created an online self-assessment to find out your Hormone Type.

You'll find it here: https://drcorinadunlap.com/assessment/.

You'll answer a series of questions about your health history, recurring patterns you notice in your life, symptoms you want to address, and more. After doing the assessment, the results will be emailed to you. You'll receive your results based on how closely you align with each type. For instance, you might score 80%

Achiever, 15% Caretaker, and 5% Survivor. This means that Achiever is your primary Hormone Type.

Why These Types Are Helpful

What you believe determines your behavior (the behaviors you do repeatedly form ingrained patterns), and these patterns shape your health. Each Hormone Type represents a different type of woman—a woman with certain beliefs that lead to actions, which lead to outcomes.

To provide one example, Caretakers tend to believe that "my value as a human being is determined by how much I can give to others." This belief (which she may or may not even be conscious of) drives her behavior, day in, day out. She might skip breakfast because she's so busy caring for her family, which leads to a blood sugar crash, which sends her body into survival mode, which sets off a ricochet of hormonal imbalances (insulin, glucagon, cortisol, and others) that can lead to a wide range of health issues, from insomnia to infertility and beyond.

What sets the negative snowball in motion? First and foremost, her *beliefs*. What a woman believes about the world shapes her choices and, ultimately, the length and quality of her life.

Beliefs aren't the *only* factors that influence your health, of course. Other factors, such as environmental toxins and genetics, also play a role (something we will discuss in future chapters). But your beliefs are a significant factor, and unlike family history, they are something you can change.

This is why knowing your Hormone Type is very helpful information. As you read Part Two, you'll meet each Hormone Type and learn how she thinks, her tendencies and patterns, and the hormonal ramifications that ensue.

Knowing your Hormone Type helps you to understand yourself better: the core beliefs that drive your behavior. Why you do certain things. Why you have trouble changing certain habits.

And, how you can retrain your body and mind to adopt a new perspective—one that serves you, rather than harming you.

Knowing and Doing Are Not the Same Thing

Once, a medical colleague confessed to me, "I have many patients with type 2 diabetes. I tell them exactly how they need to change their eating habits to reverse this disease. They listen, and they really want to do it. But once they leave my office, they have so much trouble changing their habits. I don't know how to help them."

Her patients *know* what to do but still aren't doing it.

Meanwhile, at my clinic, I'm proud to say I've had very good success helping women change their lifestyle habits in a sustained, long-lasting way. I believe my success is largely due to my understanding of the three Hormone Types.

During my first conversation with a new patient, I can usually tell which type she is, and then I confirm my hunch with an assessment and lab testing. Once I know her Hormone Type, it gives me insight into how her mind works, which informs what I say to her and how I phrase it. (Knowing her type also provides clues about what may be happening in her body and helps me to identify sneaky issues that don't always show up on lab tests.)

I can tell a woman, "You should eat more protein throughout the day to stabilize glucose levels and prevent insulin resistance." But, if she is going to shift from *knowing* to *doing,* we first have to understand the invisible wiring of her mind and what led to her situation in the first place to change the pattern.

Wellness Is Not One Size Fits All

Here's another reason why it's helpful to know your Hormone Type: it allows you to customize your Hormone Action Plan, making it even more effective. This is essential because the wellness plan that leads to incredibly positive changes for one woman may not help another or can even be counterproductive.

For instance, if you're a Survivor (a Hormone Type that tends to struggle with sluggish digestion, weight gain, and depression), the plan I recommend for you is not going to look the same as for an Achiever (a Hormone Type that often over-exercises, underfuels, pushes herself to the point of exhaustion, and struggles to slow down and rest).

All three types can achieve optimal health—a state of flourishing vitality, where all systems in the body are functioning well, hormone levels are in the optimal range, and you feel *amazing*. However, the path to get there will be different depending on your type.

We're All Alike (and Different)

Every woman, regardless of her Hormone Type, needs seven to nine hours of high-quality sleep each night. Every woman needs nutritious food and fresh water. Every woman's body is designed to move. There are universal wellness principles that apply to every type. However, based on your type, you can fine-tune your Hormone Action Plan and make it more specific and effective for you.

Throughout Parts Two and Three, I'll show you ways to personalize your Hormone Action Plan depending on your type. Customization is what makes the difference between a wellness plan that sort of works and one that *really* works.

Know Your Type—and Collaborate with Your Team

The Hormone Type Assessment is a tool that I hope you'll use and enjoy.[1] Like any powerful tool, it should be used responsibly and with appropriate support. I recommend meeting with a naturopathic doctor (or another provider) to discuss your Hormone Type and Hormone Action Plan and to get their input. I typically recommend lab testing to establish a baseline of your hormone levels now, as well as follow-up testing to confirm that your wellness plan is working and that the desired changes are occurring.

Next: go online to do the assessment, find out your type, and I'll meet you in the next chapter!

https://drcorinadunlap.com/assessment/

Note

1. It goes without saying, but I will go ahead and say it anyway: the Hormone Type Assessment is an educational resource, not a replacement for medical care. It should be used alongside other tools, like lab testing and care from a licensed professional, rather than instead of.

Chapter 3

The Caretaker

Annie had two children in the span of three years. The first was planned. The second was a surprise. Once she recovered from the initial shock of an unexpected pregnancy, she and her husband began looking forward to their new arrival. It wasn't the ideal timing (they had hoped to wait a few years before expanding their family), but it was exciting nonetheless.

The pregnancy was relatively smooth and uneventful. But then, after a frightening birth experience that ended with an emergency C-section, the new baby was taken to the neonatal intensive care unit (NICU). Annie was dazed and stunned.

Fast-forward three months. . .Annie, her toddler, and her infant are all back at home. Because her husband has a demanding job that requires long days (and sometimes late nights) away from the house, Annie is mostly alone with the two little ones, often for 12–16 hours straight with no breaks, in addition to nursing throughout the night.

On the surface, it looks like Annie is doing okay. She is recovering well from her C-section, at least physically. She is busy and active. Cleaning the house. Changing endless diapers. Walking the dog. Costco runs to stock the kitchen. Prepping meals. All the things.

Although she is performing all the tasks that need to be done, internally she is not okay. What nobody aside from her therapist knows is that she has been experiencing overwhelming anxiety. Intrusive thoughts. Feelings of panic and doom. Mostly, these thoughts center around dying. "What if my husband dies?" "What if I die?" "What would happen to the kids?" As these terrifying thoughts escalate, Annie struggles to breathe. She feels as though her chest is tightening up, like something is squeezing her heart, and then she wonders, "Maybe I *am* dying?" Her anxious thoughts spiral around and around, until it's hard to remember which came first. The scary thoughts or the physical symptoms?

Annie is an example of the Caretaker type. She is the supermom. The giver. The helper. The multitasker. The one who prioritizes everyone else's needs above her own. The woman juggling 100 balls in the air, except for one: her own well-being.

How the Caretaker Presents

Caretakers are not always mothers, but they often perform caregiving roles in some capacity. This can look like caring for children, elderly parents, or other loved ones. It can also look like tending to the needs of clients, patients, customers, students, or a team at work.

The Caregiver can present as:

An exhausted **mom** who struggles with anxious ruminating thoughts, worries, or insecurities.	An overworking **manager** who gives excessively to her team at work, picking up the slack when her colleagues don't follow through.	A busy **freelancer** who cares deeply about her clients but struggles to enforce boundaries.
"Did I remember to double-check the child lock on the bathroom cabinet. . . ."	*"It's okay, I'll just handle it myself. . . ."*	*"Even though it's the weekend, I'll just get it done. . . ."*

For the Caretaker, "I have so much to do. . ." is a constant refrain in her head.

Polished—At Least on the Surface

Like Annie, the Caretaker often appears to have all her ducks in a row. She may appear capable and productive, and she is. However, the Caretaker frequently struggles internally in ways that aren't obvious or visible to others. Anxiety. Spinning thoughts. Sleep issues. Stomach pain.

She performs a great deal of invisible labor for others, the unseen and often underappreciated work of parenting, domestic tasks, and emotional caregiving.

I'm not sure people really see or understand just how much I do every day, she may think to herself. Her contributions feel invisible. Her pain is often invisible, too. She may not always show visible signs of distress or disease, like an inflamed rash or extreme weight loss. People in her life may not realize that she is "not doing okay." And the Caretaker may choose to keep her issues private rather than asking for help, not wanting to "burden" others with her pain.

Even when she senses that something is "off" with her body, the Caretaker often pushes through it, saying to herself, *I have to keep going. So many people depend on me.* By ignoring her own needs and muscling through to the next item on her to-do list, the Caretaker sinks lower on a scale that I call the Wellness Spectrum.

The Wellness Spectrum

Imagine a spectrum running from 0 on the left to 10 on the right with 0 being extreme distress and 10 being optimal health.

A 0 represents a woman who is severely depleted and dysregulated, to the point where her life is in immediate peril. She may even have a debilitating disease or be in extreme distress. Life no longer holds joy or meaning. Her body feels like a prison that she wants to escape.

A 10 represents a woman who is flourishing and thriving. Her hormone levels are in the optimal ranges. All her bodily systems, such as endocrine system, digestive system, reproductive system, cardiovascular system, nervous system, etc., are functioning in the ideal manner. She looks and feels incredible, emanating radiant health and vitality. (Reaching a 10 on the Wellness Spectrum doesn't mean "perfect health" or being "100% disease-free." This level of perfection does not exist. What 10 means is that you feel vibrant, and any chronic conditions you may have are well-managed and causing minimal to no distress.)

Annie, the mom of two that I introduced earlier, is currently sitting at a 3 or 4 on the Wellness Spectrum. Her hormones are out of balance. Her nutrients are depleted. She is wired but tired. Various organs and systems are being impacted. Her mental health is deteriorating. A negative snowball effect has begun.

Although Annie is still "functioning" and able to carry out her daily tasks, for now, if things don't change soon, the negative snowball will gain more momentum. If left unattended, her health will sink to a 1 or 2 on the spectrum. As a naturopathic physician, my goal is to help Annie move from her current position on the Wellness Spectrum up to a 5, 6, 7, 8, and eventually all the way to 10.

Every Hormone Type—the Caretaker, Achiever, and Survivor—has the capacity to reach 10 on the Wellness Spectrum. All three types can experience radiant, flourishing health. But getting a woman to 10 requires looking at the beliefs, behaviors, and patterns that knocked her down to a lower number in the first place. Each Hormone Type has distinct tendencies and deficiencies that often arise, which is why the wellness plan I prescribe will vary depending on a woman's Hormone Type.

You Might Be a Caretaker If. . .

- You are highly sensitive and aware of other people's feelings, thoughts, and needs.
- You want everyone around you to be happy, healthy, and thriving, and give a great deal of your energy to others.

- You have trouble unwinding at the end of the day and often feel "wired but tired."
- It's difficult to turn your brain "off," even in the evenings, on weekends, or while on vacation.
- You lie awake at night replaying the day's events in your head and ruminating/thinking/fretting/worrying about what needs to happen tomorrow.
- Incoming information (an unpleasant email, distressing text, or upsetting news story) can derail you for hours, or even a whole day. It takes you quite a while to feel settled and steady again.
- Because you care so much and give so much, your mind is often preoccupied with a thousand different thoughts like "I need to do that first thing tomorrow morning" or "I have to email her back right away" or "I should check in with him."

The Caretaker's Most Common Symptoms

Symptoms are your body's way of signaling, "Something is not right." Unpleasant symptoms are not a punishment for doing something wrong but, rather, an alert to get your attention.

When the Caretaker is at a 9 or 10 on the Wellness Spectrum, a state of optimal health, she will have very mild symptoms or none. But when she sinks down to a lower number, symptoms increase and intensify. These are the most common symptoms that appear when a Caretaker is hormonally out of balance. Not all Caretakers experience these symptoms, but many do.

Emotional Symptoms

Anxiety: Anxiety is the most prevalent emotional symptom for the Caretaker. Her anxious thoughts are often accompanied by feelings of self-doubt, comparison to others, and feeling inferior in some way. Anxiety can sometimes manifest as avoidance. For instance, if you feel anxious about car accidents, you might avoid driving. If you have anxiety about your kids accidentally drowning, you may avoid being near pools. Avoiding certain places or activities can be an expression of anxiety. Over time, this restricts the Caretaker's world, making life smaller than it needs to be.

Think you might be experiencing anxiety, but not sure? Maybe you wonder, "Am I experiencing a 'normal' amount of anxiety, or is my situation more serious and potentially something to be concerned about?"

There are validated scales, such as the Generalized Anxiety Disorder 7-item scale (GAD-7), and for the postpartum period, the Perinatal Anxiety Screening Scale (PASS). For depression, we use the Patient Health Questionnaire 9-item scale (PHQ-9), and for the postpartum period, the Edinburgh Postnatal Depression Scale (EPDS). You can use all these tools to assess yourself, or with the support of your healthcare provider, and find out if your anxiety or depression levels might be considered "minimal," mild," "moderate," or "severe." Go online and search for "GAD-7 assessment,"[1] "PASS,"[2] "EPDS,"[3] or "PHQ-9"[4] to find these evaluation tools.

Overwhelm: The Caretaker often feels overwhelmed by the sheer amount of responsibility on her shoulders. (If you've ever watched the movie *Encanto*, the character of Luisa Madrigal is a prime example of an overburdened Caretaker.)

Guilt: The Caretaker may experience pangs of guilt when she needs to step away from her responsibilities, even if it's only for a short time. Even if she takes a break to go for a walk or get a pedicure, she feels so guilty or worried the entire time that it's difficult to enjoy the experience. It feels stressful rather than restful.

Cognitive Symptoms

Difficulty concentrating: The Caretaker may or may not meet the diagnostic criteria for attention deficit hyperactivity disorder (ADHD) but presents with many of the same symptoms, including difficulty focusing for long periods of time, difficulty regulating emotions, easily distracted, and derailed by minor interruptions (such as a phone notification) and has trouble refocusing on what she was doing before.

Wondering if you meet the criteria for ADHD? Talk to your therapist or psychiatrist about doing an ADHD screening. Your provider will use the guidelines in the American Psychiatric Association's Diagnostic and Statistical Manual (DSM) to determine if what you're experiencing is ADHD or something else or perhaps (as is the case for many women) ADHD plus something else.

If you do have ADHD, it's important to know that hormonal changes can exacerbate ADHD symptoms. Some women with ADHD notice that their symptoms are more intense when their estrogen levels are lower (such as during the beginning of their menstrual cycle) and improve when estrogen is higher.[5] *Although ADHD is not "caused" by hormonal imbalances, ADHD and hormones are very much intertwined.*

Physical Symptoms

When a Caretaker comes into my clinic, often her chronically elevated stress levels have led to adrenal and thyroid dysfunction.

Disrupted ovulation: She may be having regular periods but not ovulating every cycle. She may even be at risk for early perimenopausal symptoms and early menopause.

Energy crashes: Because she tends to skip meals or eat poorly while rushing around tending to others, she often struggles with blood sugar spikes and crashes.

Sleep issues: She often has difficulty falling asleep or wakes up at 3 or 4 a.m. feeling wide awake (another indicator of adrenal issues). When Caretakers come into my clinic, they often tell me: "I feel exhausted." "I haven't had a good night's sleep in so long." "My physician prescribed sleep medication, but I'd like to get off it."

Nervous System Wiring: Safety and Threats for the Caretaker

Your nervous system (which includes your brain, spinal cord, and a network of nerves throughout your body) has an important job: scanning your surroundings for potential threats to your safety.

Threats can be physical. For example, a fire in the building, an aggressive dog running toward you, a bicyclist that's about to crash into you, or another threat to your physical well-being. Threats can also be psychological. For instance, a boss or client who is unhappy with your work, a spouse who seems distant or cold, or something that causes you to feel cast out, isolated, or emotionally vulnerable.

When your nervous system detects a potential threat, it signals your body to produce certain hormones, including adrenaline (epinephrine), noradrenaline (norepinephrine), and cortisol. These chemical messengers rapidly prepare your body to respond, raising heart rate and blood pressure, sharpening alertness, mobilizing blood sugar, and shifting resources away from long-term processes like digestion, reproduction, and repair.

The nervous system's job is to protect you from danger and keep you alive. This is a critical role. However, the nervous system's focus on self-preservation can also be counterproductive, interfering with your well-being. This plays out differently for women, depending on their Hormone Type.

The Caretaker believes, "My value as a human being is determined by what I can give to others." By giving to others, often excessively, she secures her sense of safety. Her sense of safety is threatened when she perceives, "I am no longer needed or valuable to the people around me." This is why, for the Caretaker, the idea of stepping away from her responsibilities for a week, a day, or even an hour can feel extremely uncomfortable. Yet, for the Caretaker, this is precisely what she needs more than anything, to step back from caregiving for others and begin caring more for herself.

To achieve optimal health, the Caretaker must retrain her nervous system to recognize a new kind of safety, which means adopting a new set of beliefs: "I am safe even when I have to set boundaries. I am safe even when I can't complete my to-do list. I am safe even when I choose to put myself first."

Just like you can rewire the electrical system in your home, you can rewire your nervous system to perceive safety in a different way. Though it's not always easy, you can build new beliefs. Doing this often requires coaching, therapy, or both, and a firm commitment to changing patterns in your life.

For the Caretaker, and for all Hormone Types, achieving flourishing wellness, a 10 on the Wellness Spectrum, often requires doing the one thing that feels the most threatening and uncomfortable. For Caretakers, whatever you are resisting most is putting yourself first; this is what will create the biggest transformation.

The Caretaker		
Safety	**Threat**	**Shift**
She feels safe when she perceives: "I am needed by others and valuable to those around me."	She feels unsafe when she perceives: "I am no longer needed or valuable."	She achieves optimal wellness when she shifts to a new set of beliefs: "I can prioritize my *own* needs, not just the needs of others, and *still* feel safe."

What's Happening on a Biomedical Level

When the Caretaker Is Not Well: First, Second, and Third Levels of Impact

Your body includes 11 distinct systems, including the cardiovascular, digestive, lymphatic, reproductive, immune, and nervous systems, to name a few. When a Caretaker's hormones get out of whack and she begins sinking lower on the Wellness Spectrum, out of these 11 systems, it's her *nervous system* that is impacted first.

To reverse the negative trend and start feeling better, she needs to bring attention to restoring her nervous system first and foremost. As the negative snowball gains momentum, and her nervous system begins to buckle under the strain, her adrenals, thyroid, and ovaries are impacted second. *Gut health* is likely to suffer, too, as the third level of impact.

Why is this important to understand? When a Caretaker client comes into my clinic, if she's experiencing late-stage adrenal dysregulation, thyroid issues, ovarian dysfunction, *and* digestive issues too, that's a clue that her hormonal dysregulation has likely been going on for quite some time, because we have reached the tertiary level of impact. Knowing this, I might recommend a more aggressive treatment plan compared to a Caretaker whose situation hasn't advanced that far yet. See Figure 3.1.

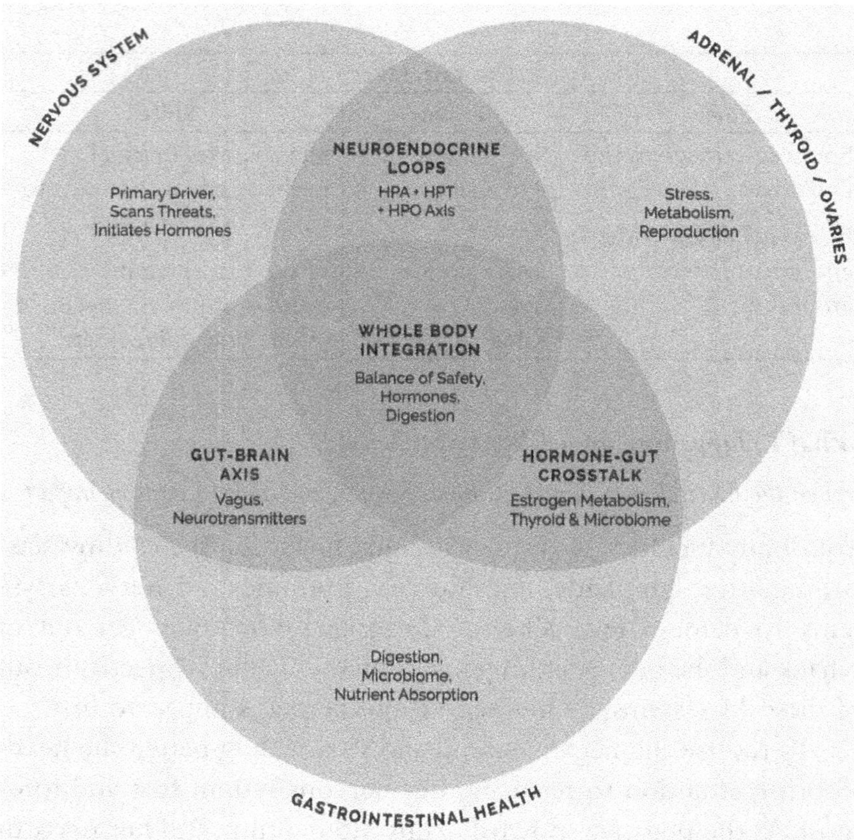

Figure 3.1 Nervous system and interconnected systems.

When the Nervous System Rules: A Physiologic Cascade

Let's look closer at how the cascade from the Caretaker's nervous system to adrenals to thyroid, and ovaries to gastrointestinal health, plays out.

Primary Driver: Nervous System Overactivation

For the Caretaker, the nervous system is the dominant influence in her body. This system branches into two subsystems: the parasympathetic and sympathetic nervous systems.

Parasympathetic: Often called the "rest and digest" system, or the "feed and breed" system. This system is engaged when your nervous system perceives, "I am safe; it's okay to relax." You feel calm, at ease, and when this system is highly engaged, even drowsy. Imagine the way you feel when you're reading peacefully in a cozy nook, listening to a soothing meditation, or drifting off to sleep. That's parasympathetic energy. It says, "Slow down and relax."

Sympathetic: This is the "fight or flight" system that is mobilized when your body perceives a potential threat. When engaged, you get a temporary surge of energy due to hormones such as adrenaline, noradrenaline, and cortisol. Again, this energy spike is useful during a life-threatening emergency. But it's not something you want happening too often, because it takes a heavy toll on the body. Imagine the way you feel when you're sprinting to snatch a baby's hand away from an uncovered electrical socket. This is sympathetic energy. It says, "Speed up and GO!"

Parasympathetic Nervous System	**Sympathetic Nervous System**
Engaged when: Your body perceives safety. "I'm safe. It's okay to rest and relax."	*Engaged when:* Your body perceives a threat. "I'm not safe. Danger!"

Parasympathetic Nervous System	**Sympathetic Nervous System**
Primary neurotransmitter associated with this system: Acetylcholine.	*Primary neurotransmitters and hormones associated with this system:* Adrenaline, noradrenaline, and cortisol.
When activated, you feel: Secure, calm and relaxed, connected to others, unguarded.	*When activated, you feel:* Aggressive, mobilized for action, high energy, defensive, primed to attack or flee.

Caretakers often experience *sympathetic overdrive*. This means the sympathetic nervous system has been working too hard, for too long. When this system remains switched on for months or years, it reprograms your physiology in the following ways:

- *HPA axis hyperactivation*, which leads to cortisol dysregulation (initially, cortisol levels are too high; later, we see flattened rhythms)
- *Autonomic imbalance*, which leads to vagal withdrawal (the vagus nerve is the longest nerve in your nervous system), reducing gut motility, digestion, and microbiome resilience
- *Neuroendocrine disruption*, which impairs GnRH pulsatility, disrupts ovarian hormone signaling

The Caretaker's impaired nervous system, strained from sympathetic overdrive, sets off a chain reaction in the adrenals, thyroid, ovaries, and gut.

Secondary Impact: Adrenals, Thyroid, and Ovaries

When stress is unremitting, the adrenals, thyroid, and ovaries act as shock absorbers for nervous system overdrive.

- ***Adrenals:*** Cortisol elevations suppress GnRH pulsatility, impair ovulation, increase visceral fat deposition, and dysregulate circadian sleep/wake cycles.

Over time, the Caretaker's labs may show:

- Elevated morning cortisol (early stage), which leads to a flattened diurnal, or daytime, curve (later stage).
- DHEA decline (DHEA, or dehydroepiandrosterone, is a hormone that is a precursor to testosterone and estrogen, and when DHEA is too low, your body is less resilient when it comes to handling stress and fighting off illnesses.)

- ***Thyroid:*** Stress hormones alter TSH secretion, reduce peripheral T4→T3 conversion, and increase reverse T3 as an energy-conserving adaptation. Labs may reveal:
  - Subclinical hypothyroidism (TSH > 2.5–4.5 mIU/L)
  - Low free T3, often elevated reverse T3

- ***Ovaries:*** Chronic cortisol signaling disrupts follicle development and ovulation, lowers luteal phase progesterone, and accelerates ovarian aging. Labs may reflect:
  - Low luteal progesterone.
  - Short luteal phase or anovulatory cycles (tracked via LH, mid-luteal progesterone, or cycle mapping).
  - Declining anti-Müllerian hormone (AMH/ovarian reserve) earlier than expected in some women.

As the adrenals, thyroid, and ovaries suffer, this cascades into the next level of impact:

Tertiary Impact: Gastrointestinal Health

Chronic sympathetic dominance (aka sympathetic overdrive) shuts down the body's ability to "rest and digest." In other words, as your sympathetic system over-fires, your parasympathetic system atrophies and becomes less effective. It becomes harder and harder to relax, recharge, and recover.

- *Hypochlorhydria* (low stomach acid), which leads to malabsorption and can lead to deficiencies including iron, zinc, and B12.

- *Dysbiosis* (imbalance in the gut microbiome), which leads to decreased microbial diversity, leaky gut, and digestive systemic inflammation.
- This results in *IBS-like symptoms* (bloating, irregular bowel movements).

Lab findings may include:

- Low ferritin, B12, and vitamin D
- Elevated inflammatory markers (CRP, calprotectin)
- Reduced microbial diversity in stool samples
- Pathogenic or opportunistic gut infections

Decade by Decade: How the Negative Snowball Rolls

If you're a Caretaker and your hormones are off, here's an example of how the negative snowball tends to build momentum through the decades (see Figure 3.2):

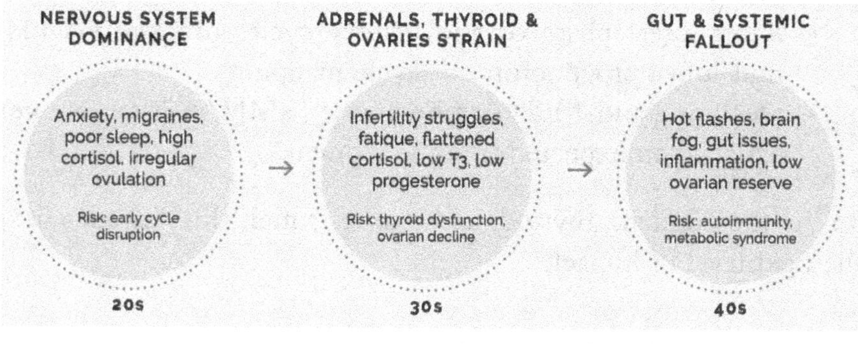

Figure 3.2 Progression of nervous system dominance across decades.

20s: Nervous System Sets the Tone

- *Symptoms:* Anxiety, migraines, heart palpitations, feeling "wired but tired"
- *Labs reveal:* High AM cortisol, irregular LH surges, occasional anovulation
- *Risks:* Early cycle irregularity, iron deficiency, subclinical hypothyroid patterns (fatigue, hair loss, slowed digestion, bloating, dry skin)

30s: Adrenals, Thyroid, and Ovaries Bear the Burden

- *Symptoms:* Infertility struggles, irregular cycles, unusually light or heavy or anovulatory bleeding, fatigue
- *Labs reveal:* Flattened cortisol curve, declining DHEA, high/normal TSH, low free T3, elevated reverse T3, low luteal progesterone, and early Hashimoto's antibodies in some, high/normal blood glucose levels
- *Risks:* Subclinical hypothyroidism, diminished ovarian reserve, insulin resistance, postpartum depression/anxiety

40s: Gastrointestinal and Systemic Fallout

- *Symptoms:* Hot flashes, night sweats, stubborn weight gain, brain fog, IBS symptoms, and autoimmune flare
- *Labs reveal:* Low ovarian reserve markers (AMH, FSH elevation), persistent suboptimal thyroid labs, and inflammatory markers up (hs-CRP, ferritin, cytokines)
- *Risks:* Early or difficult perimenopause, metabolic syndrome, weight gain, autoimmunity, and mood disorders

Symptoms Become Conditions

Without intervention, the trajectory for a Caretaker can shift from invisible labor and invisible symptoms to diagnosable disease states. When left unattended, over time:

- Anxiety can become generalized anxiety disorder or a panic disorder.
- Disrupted ovulation can escalate into infertility or premature ovarian insufficiency.
- Fatigue/thyroid dysfunction can become hypothyroidism or Hashimoto's thyroiditis.
- Gut dysbiosis can turn into IBS, IBD, or an autoimmune disorder.
- Metabolic strain may eventually lead to insulin resistance and prediabetes.

The good news? Symptoms can be addressed, and most conditions are reversible. With the right plan and some patience, a distressed Caretaker can transform into a thriving woman.

The Flourishing Caretaker

We've spent some time discussing what happens when the Caretaker is *not* well. But what about the other end of the spectrum? What is the highest potential for a Caretaker? This section discusses what I have witnessed in my practice.

When a Caretaker reaches a 10 on the Wellness Spectrum, she is a role model who gives generously to others while giving just as generously to herself. A vibrant caregiver, not a depleted one. She is extraordinary in whatever role she chooses. Her mindset has shifted, and she now believes, "I'm doing a disservice to others when I neglect myself. Putting myself first is a gift to myself and everyone I care about."

Because of this new belief, she exhibits new behaviors. She might wake up before the kids to have some quiet time for herself in the early morning, not to meal prep or "get a head start" on chores, but to enjoy a moment of stillness. She eats breakfast rather than skipping or forgetting. She books that well-deserved massage and actually *enjoys* the experience, rather than fretting that she ought to be elsewhere. New beliefs lead to new behaviors, which become new patterns, which alter her physiology, restoring balance and resulting in new health outcomes.

A flourishing Caregiver is aware of her own tendencies. Even at a 10 on the Wellness Spectrum, she is still human. She is not perfect. She sometimes struggles to put herself first and make her own needs a priority. When she notices herself backsliding into old habits, such as neglecting her health, goals, or dreams, and overgiving to others, she catches things quickly. The flourishing Caretaker course-corrects right away before the negative snowball gains too much momentum.

What the Caretaker Needs Most

How can the Caretaker attain a 10 on the Wellness Spectrum and feel incredible? To get there, what should the Caretaker focus on first?

First and foremost, if you're a Caretaker, your primary assignment is to put yourself at the top of your to-do list, finding a balance between serving others and pouring into your own cup.

If you're a Caretaker, prioritizing yourself may feel uncomfortable at first, like you're breaking a deeply ingrained pattern, because that's exactly what you're doing. Disrupting the status quo. This may feel scary, but it's the "good" kind of scary. Deep down, the wisest part of you knows, "I know this is what I need to do, even though it's unfamiliar."

As you do this, you'll notice that many symptoms you have been experiencing (anxious thoughts, difficulty concentrating, sleep issues, and others) begin to subside. They may not vanish completely, but you may notice a slight improvement, which then makes it easier to make other changes in your life. The negative snowball begins to switch direction, becoming a positive one.

My Hormone Type is the Caretaker, so the advice I just laid out is the advice I repeatedly give myself.

While writing this book, my Caretaker patterns kept creeping in. I found it incredibly difficult to concentrate on writing because, "My kids need me," "I have to reply to patient messages right away," "My team at the clinic needs me to pop in," or "My husband is so supportive, but I don't want to ask him to do too much."

Even when I decided to go on a writing retreat in Hawaii (four days of quiet time and space to finally focus on writing the book!), my Caretaker tendencies kept creeping in. I felt guilty for being in such a beautiful, luxurious setting while my husband was handling all the parenting duties back at home. Guilty for soaking in the jacuzzi under the stars. Guilty for taking time to get a massage. Guilty for focusing on writing rather than my other duties and responsibilities. Guilty for not writing "fast enough."

"Oh, let me help you with that!" I blurted out when the retreat host cleared away my dishes after a meal, to which she replied, "It's okay, go relax, let me take care of this."

For a Caretaker like me, who is accustomed to caring for others and derives great purpose from doing so, being the recipient of care, rather than the giver, can feel unsettling and even create a deep sense of guilt. Many women who work in healing and helping professions—teachers, nurses, doctors, nonprofit leaders—are, not surprisingly, Caretaker types.

On that retreat, I reminded myself, **"The very thing I am resisting is the very thing I need most."**

When the Caretaker focuses on her own well-being before assisting others, it supports her hormonal health. It's what steers her toward optimal health. It's what unleashes her greatest work into the world, whether that work involves raising kids, building a business, becoming an author, or anything else. It's what closes the gap between the life she has now and the one she wants to have. Though it may feel threatening at first, over time, with practice, caring for herself does become easier.

If your Hormone Type is the Caretaker, **how could you pour into your own cup today?**

Key Takeaways

- The three Hormone Types are the Caretaker, the Achiever, and the Survivor.
- The Caretaker tends to expend a great deal of energy caring for others (children, elders, clients, students, etc.), and she often neglects her own needs in the process.
- Over time, deprioritizing herself causes hormonal imbalances, which, if unattended, builds up into a negative snowball that gathers strength and speed through the decades.

- The Caretaker often performs a lot of invisible labor—the unseen work of parenting, domestic tasks, and emotional caregiving. Many of her initial symptoms are invisible, too.
- When out of balance, the most common emotional symptoms for a Caretaker are anxiety, overwhelm, and guilt.
- The most common cognitive symptom is difficulty concentrating.
- Common physical symptoms include disrupted ovulation, energy crashes, and sleep issues.
- When she is hormonally dysregulated, the Caretaker's nervous system is the first system to suffer under the strain. Second, her adrenals, thyroid, and ovaries are impacted. The third level of impact is her gastrointestinal health.
- To turn the negative snowball into a positive one, the Caretaker's assignment is to make *herself* a top priority rather than an afterthought.
- At first, this can be unsettling for the Caretaker and can even feel threatening to her nervous system. But over time, her nervous system can be retrained and rewired to this new reality.
- No matter your Hormone Type, to achieve flourishing health, your assignment is to do the very thing you have been resisting the most.

Notes

1. "GAD-7 Anxiety." Anxiety & Depression Association of America. ADAA. 2025. https://adaa.org/sites/default/files/GAD-7_Anxiety-updated_0.pdf.
2. Somerville, S., et al. (2014). The Perinatal Anxiety Screening Scale: Development and Preliminary Validation. *Archives of Women's Mental Health*, 17, 443–454. https://doi.org/10.1007/s00737-014-0425-8.

3. https://www.mdcalc.com/calc/10466/edinburgh-postnatal-depression-scale-epds.
4. https://wwaw.mdcalc.com/calc/1725/phq9-patient-health-questionnaire9.
5. "Those Lovely 'Mones: The Intersection of ADHD and Hormones." Attention Magazine. Linda Roggli. 2021. https://chadd.org/adhd-news/adhd-news-adults/attention-those-lovely-mones-the-intersection-of-adhd-and-hormones/.

Chapter 4

The Achiever

Regina is the founder and chief executive officer (CEO) of a massively successful company, which she built with her own blood, sweat, tears, and personal savings, with no assistance from outside investors. Prior to starting her own company, back when she worked in corporate, she was always praised for being a "top performer" and an "asset to the company," frequently securing promotions, raises, and bonuses for her achievements.

A lifelong athlete, Regina has completed several marathons and plans on doing an ultramarathon in the future. She loves doing what others might consider impossible, in business, in athletics, in all aspects of life. Pushing beyond her current limits gives her a rush of excitement. She is, by her own admission, "extremely driven" and a "classic Type A personality." With any goal that she sets, failure is unacceptable. Simply "trying" is not good enough, either. She wants to *win*.

Her body is lean and sculpted, reflecting someone who is exceptionally disciplined with her diet and exercise regimen. On the outside, she looks like a model from the cover of *Women's Fitness* magazine. But inside? It's a different story.

During one of our first conversations, Regina tells me about her fertility struggles. After trying to conceive naturally for two years, to no avail, she and her partner decided to pursue in vitro fertilization (IVF). But after several embryo transfers that didn't work out—her uterine lining rejected the embryos and wouldn't retain them—she came to me, frustrated and looking for new options to try.

As we discussed her medical history, Regina's grief and discouragement began to seep through. Her eyes welled with tears, and her voice shook as she shared how much she wanted to be a mother.

"At this point," she told me, "I am open to trying anything you might suggest."

I could almost hear the unspoken words in her head:

> "I always achieve whatever I set out to do. So why am I struggling to get pregnant? Other women get pregnant all the time, sometimes by accident, without even trying! So, why is this not happening for me?"

Like many of my patients, Regina's Hormone Type is the Achiever. When in optimal health, the Achiever is an unstoppable force. But while her drive to succeed is a strength, it also has a shadow side and can become the very thing that derails her health.

How the Achiever Presents

I've met plenty of Achievers who lead a more sedentary lifestyle, and their achievement-oriented personality shows up in other ways. For instance, an Achiever might work nonstop and drive extraordinary results for her organization, at the expense of her own health. She might be extremely accomplished in one area of life and neglect another entirely.

Out of the three Hormone Types—Caretaker, Achiever, and Survivor—the Achiever is the one that struggles the most with moderation and balance.

The Achiever can present as:

A **corporate** attorney who is on the partner track—and putting in brutal 80-hour work weeks to get there.	A stay-at-home mom who is extremely **goal-oriented and perfectionistic** and wants to be "the best" in everything she does.	Someone who has been an exceptional athlete their whole life and has transitioned this **competitive push** to all areas of life.

The Achiever is often attracted to extremes: extremely demanding sports, extremely restrictive clean eating, extremely high standards. Or she may be highly dedicated to a specific wellness protocol for a while but then abandon it because it's too restrictive or didn't work well enough, as her body pushes back against the extreme adherence.

The Achiever struggles with taking a moderate approach. For her, life tends to be all-or-nothing. There is success, there is failure, and there is no gray area in between. She is proactive, competitive, a go-getter, and tends to push her body and mind to the absolute limit.

By pushing too hard, for too long, without resting and refueling adequately to support such intense output, the Achiever sinks lower on the Wellness Spectrum.

The Wellness Spectrum

To refresh your memory, on the Wellness Spectrum, 0 indicates extreme distress and 10 indicates optimal health.

As I mentioned in the prior chapter, being at a 10 doesn't necessarily mean being 100% disease-free or feeling amazing 100% of the time. You can have a chronic condition or be in recovery from a serious illness and still be at a 10 on the Wellness Spectrum. A 10 means you are thriving overall, your symptoms have diminished significantly, and you feel little to no distress.

Achievers, just like Caretakers and Survivors, can reach a 10 on the Wellness Spectrum. Because Achievers are so goal-oriented, they often feel confused or even angry when their health is anything less than "perfect."

You Might Be an Achiever If. . .

- You are incredibly focused and driven. A doer. A finisher. The one who makes it happen.
- You tend to overdo it. Overworking. Overdelivering. Overexercising. Overextending in many ways.
- You work all day and forget to eat. Or drink coffee all day and forget to drink water.
- You swing to extremes when it comes to food, movement, and other habits—it's either CrossFit six times a week or no exercise at all. A totally clean diet or overindulging in junk food. Black and white. All or nothing.
- You push until you literally can't push anymore—and then your body forces you to slow down due to an injury, illness, severe burnout, etc.
- You ignore the inner whispers from your body saying, "Rest more," "Slow down," or "Hey, I need this. . .," and eventually those whispers become a shout.

The Achiever's Most Common Symptoms

Symptoms are your body's way of signaling, "Something is not right." When you experience an unpleasant symptom, whether it's acne, bloating, weight gain, low mood, chronic infections, or anything else, think of it as a text message alert from your body, letting you know, "Hey, something is off and needs your attention."

When the Achiever is at a 9 or 10 on the Wellness Spectrum—a state of optimal health—she will have few to no symptoms, and/or those symptoms will be mild. But when she sinks to a lower number, these are the most common symptoms that appear. Not all Achievers experience these symptoms, but many do.

Emotional Symptoms

Volatile self-esteem: When the Achiever is "winning," she tends to feel good about herself—at least, for a brief time. But when she feels not as successful as she could be, her positive outlook quickly turns to despair. Although she may appear confident to others, her self-esteem is fickle. How she feels about herself depends on external metrics of success, which may fluctuate up and down, rather than being derived from within. She may experience interpersonal dependence, reflecting a greater need for approval and praise from others.

Hypercritical tendencies: The Achiever holds herself to very high standards, sometimes impossibly high. Pursuing perfection, which is never attainable, leaves her feeling "not good enough." She is hypercritical of herself and often feels dissatisfied or discouraged when she doesn't do things "perfectly." The relentless pursuit of "more," "better," "faster" makes it difficult for her to celebrate and appreciate everything she has already achieved.

Heightened need for control: "If I do X, then I get Y" is the Achiever's motto. She craves a feeling of control. She likes when things feel straightforward and linear: *do the action, get the desired result.* She has little tolerance for uncertainty. Behaviorally, this can show up as micromanaging, rigidity, difficulty delegating, or tremendous discomfort when matters are not within her control. This is why certain experiences, such as trying to conceive or being pregnant, can be especially challenging for the Achiever. Not having a guaranteed outcome is terrifying for her. Surrender and "going with the flow" do not come easily to Achiever types.

Cognitive Symptoms

Cognitive inflexibility: The Achiever often exhibits rigid thinking patterns and heightened concern about others' judgments, as well as a negative self-perception when she doesn't adhere to her self-imposed standards. This rigidity is more pronounced, especially if she has a suppressed period, more so than in women with regular menstrual cycles. This is because when the hormones that dictate your cycle are off, they can affect other organs and glands throughout your body, including those that produce mood-stabilizing hormones.

Difficulty coping with stress: The Achiever can have trouble managing daily stressors and reduced coping abilities, which may present as overfixation on tasks or despair when things don't go their way.

Depressive symptoms: Higher levels of depressive symptoms are commonly observed in the Achiever. Whereas the Caretaker is more likely to experience anxious thoughts, the Achiever has more of a tendency toward a low or depressed mood.

Intrusive thoughts and psychological distress: Intrusive, unwanted thoughts and obsessive-compulsive traits are also frequently reported by my Achiever patients. OCD traits can include performing "rituals" (such as repeated hand washing, checking the stove to make sure it's off, or quadruple-checking documents at work) as a way of gaining temporary relief from emotional distress.

These compulsive rituals create a quick spike in dopamine levels, which feels good temporarily, but the relief doesn't last. The compulsion to "do it again" creeps in almost immediately.

Think you may have OCD? OCD is often misdiagnosed as anxiety because some of the warning signs are similar.[1] *However, these conditions are not the same, and the best practices for treating anxiety are different from the best ways to handle OCD. Visit the American Psychological Association (APA) website, or check out* TreatMyOCD.com, *to find resources about OCD and its many subtypes, as well as treatment specialists who may be covered by your insurance.*

Disordered eating: Cognitive symptoms often overlap with disordered eating behaviors, such as a strong drive for thinness, preoccupation with weight, and even preoccupation with fitness. Even if she doesn't meet the full criteria for anorexia, bulimia, or another eating disorder, she may still struggle with disordered thoughts around food or body image. Similarly, my Achiever patients may experience orthorexia, an overwhelming preoccupation with only eating "pure," "clean," or "healthy" foods, to such an extreme degree that it makes daily life distressing.

Physical Symptoms

Missing or irregular periods: Many Achievers (though not all) experience periods when their menstrual cycles are absent or irregular. Often, she doesn't recognize the profound importance of a regular cycle to her overall well-being, not because of personal oversight but because this truth hasn't been adequately emphasized by her medical providers. Instead, she is frequently offered birth control to "regulate" her cycle. Yet, research confirms that a regular menstrual cycle is a vital sign of health, linked to cardiometabolic, bone, cognitive, and reproductive well-being,[2] which is different from simply using birth control to "regulate" her cycle.

Gonadal insufficiency: When an Achiever comes into my clinic and we do lab testing, the reports often show suppressed HPG axis hormones in general, which over time leads to decreased uterine health, skin health, and brain health, low libido, bone loss (osteoporosis/osteopenia), hot flashes, and premature aging.

Nervous System Wiring: Safety and Threats for the Achiever

To briefly review what we covered in the previous chapter, your nervous system continually scans your environment, looking for potential threats. Messages travel through your brain, spinal cord, and a network of nerves throughout your body to say either "We're safe right now" or "We're not safe." Your nervous system's job is to protect you from danger. However, the nervous system's focus on self-preservation can also be counterproductive.

The Achiever believes, "My value as a human being is determined by how much I can achieve." For the Achiever, accomplishment equals success, and success equals safety. Her sense of safety is threatened when she perceives, "I am not succeeding." Not winning the athletic competition, not getting the promotion at work, not getting pregnant, or another perceived "failure" is not just disappointing for the Achiever; it is identity-shattering and profoundly unsettling to her nervous system. In the Achiever's world, winning means safety. Failing to win means, "I am not safe."

In your teens and 20s, you can pull an all-nighter to work on a project, max out your physical capacity at the gym, skimp on rest and self-care, and still function—mostly. But as you get older, this approach doesn't work all the time. Many Achievers in their 30s, 40s, and 50s feel frustrated because "the way I have always done things isn't working anymore." Their body can't tolerate the strain that it used to and begins crying out for a change.

For Achievers like Regina, one of the hardest things to do is slow down, rest, and refuel. When I encourage Regina to switch from high-intensity two-a-day workouts to gentle restorative yoga to allow her overtaxed body to recover, she blinks at me and says, "That's not going to happen."

"Dial it back." "Rest more." "Be gentle with yourself." Achievers do not like receiving this kind of advice. For an Achiever, slowing down feels like laziness, apathy, or giving up, rather than a wise and energizing choice. As much as she resists resting and taking time to refuel, this is precisely what the Achiever needs more than anything.

This often requires a rewiring of her belief system. The Achiever might currently believe: "If I slow down, I won't be successful anymore." She needs to question, "Where does this belief come from? Is it true? Is it serving me? What does 'success' mean to me? Are my current patterns bringing me there?"

It can take time and the support of a therapist, but eventually the Achiever can build a new belief system. She can eventually recognize, "Taking time to rest and restore myself actually leads to greater success than before."

For all three Hormone Types—the Caretaker, Achiever, and Survivor—achieving optimal wellness often requires doing the one thing that feels the most threatening and scary. Whatever she is resisting the most will lead to true healing.

The Achiever		
Safety	**Threat**	**Shift**
She feels safe when she perceives: "I am successfully achieving my goals."	She feels unsafe when she perceives: "I am not succeeding."	She achieves optimal wellness when she shifts to a new set of beliefs: "I am more than my accomplishments." "I can work toward my goals while taking time to rest and recharge." "I am safe even when I *don't* achieve something I intended to do."

What's Happening on a Biomedical Level

When the Achiever Is Not Well: First, Second, and Third Levels of Impact

When the Achiever's hormones are out of whack, it's her *brain* (particularly the hypothalamus and pituitary glands, both located in the base of the brain) that is negatively impacted first. For the Achiever, the brain takes center stage as the master conductor, setting the rhythm for hormone signaling and stress regulation. This is slightly different from the Caretaker, who is nervous system dominant. When the brain (hypothalamus and pituitary) is the primary driver, its hormone-releasing pulses dictate the state of the entire endocrine network.

The adrenals and ovaries are the next level of impact when the Achiever is not well, as they respond directly to brain signals to regulate stress hormones, estrogen, and progesterone. The adrenals and ovaries respond directly to pituitary signals (ACTH, LH, FSH) to regulate cortisol, estrogen, and progesterone. This is where stress response and reproductive capacity are most visible.

Thyroid and metabolic health are the third level of impact, as these rely on signals from the brain, adrenals, and ovaries to manage energy balance, weight regulation, and overall vitality. Pituitary thyroid-stimulating hormone (TSH), along with signals from the adrenals and ovaries, helps regulate energy balance, weight, and overall vitality.

When hypothalamic or pituitary signaling goes off track, all three layers destabilize in sequence: first stress/reproduction and then metabolism and long-term energy management. See Figure 4.1.

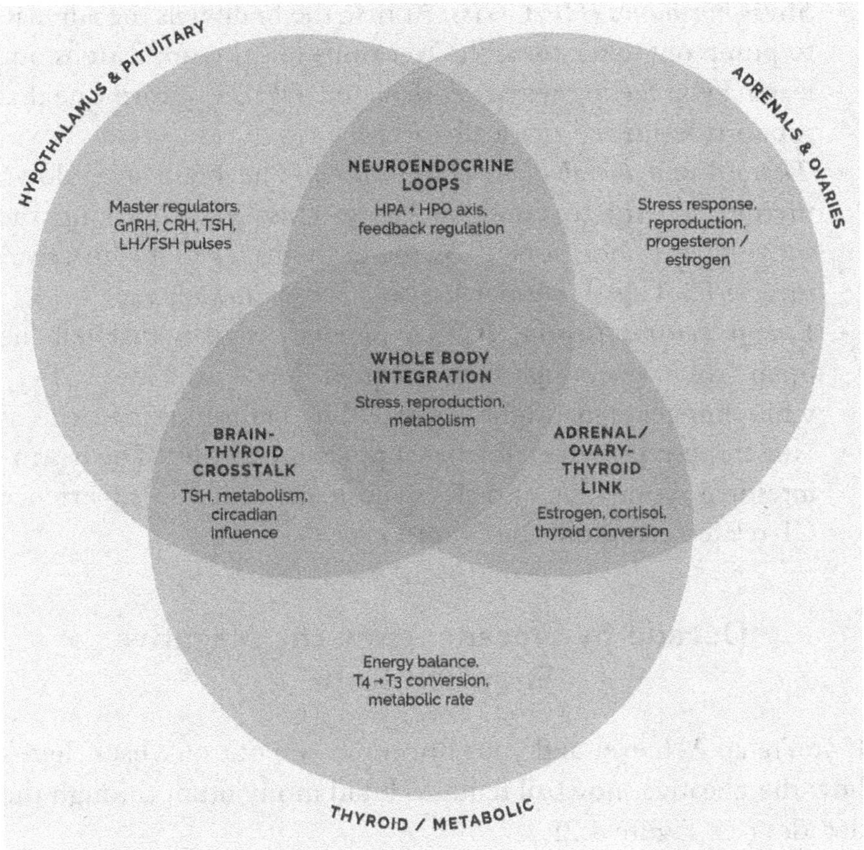

Figure 4.1 Brain (hypothalamus and pituitary) and interconnected systems.

When the Brain (Hypothalamus and Pituitary) Rules: A Physiologic Cascade

Here is how the negative snowball from the Achiever's brain to adrenals and ovaries to thyroid and metabolic health plays out.

- ***Reproductive hormones (HPG axis):*** The brain slows down its monthly signals, so ovulation becomes weak or irregular. This means lower progesterone after ovulation, thinner uterine lining, and estrogen levels that aren't quite strong enough. Fertility and cycle health both take a hit.

- ***Stress hormones (HPA axis):*** At first, the brain tells the adrenals to pump out extra cortisol. Over time, this rhythm flattens out, leaving you feeling wired yet depleted. DHEA, a hormone that supports resilience, gradually drops.
- ***Thyroid and metabolism (HPT axis):*** The brain dials down thyroid activity to conserve energy. Instead of making the active thyroid hormone (T3), the body makes more "inactive" reverse T3. This slows metabolism, energy, and repair.
- ***Energy sensors (leptin, IGF-1, ghrelin):*** Signals that tell the brain "we have enough fuel" go quiet (low leptin, low IGF-1), while hunger signals (ghrelin) rise. The brain interprets this as "unsafe to reproduce," further suppressing fertility. The gastrointestinal system can also slow, and many will also experience GI-related symptoms or conditions.

Decade by Decade: How the Negative Snowball Rolls

If you're an Achiever and your hormones are out of whack, here's how the negative snowball tends to build momentum through the decades (see Figure 4.2):

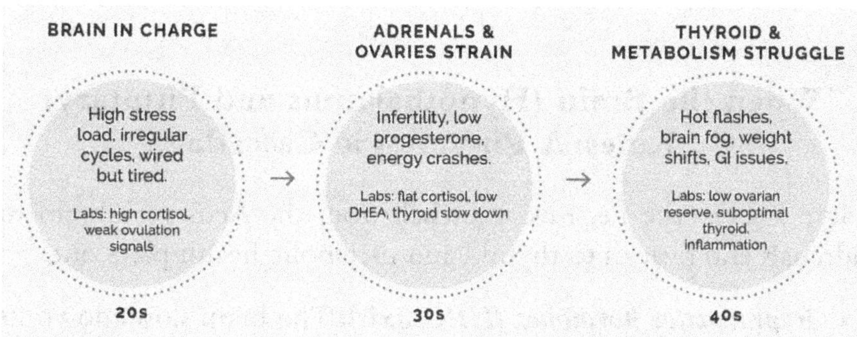

Figure 4.2 Progression across the decades: brain to adrenals/ovaries to thyroid/metabolism.

20s: Brain in Charge

- *Symptoms:* High-functioning anxiety, irregular cycles, "wired but depleted"
- *Labs reveal:* High AM cortisol; irregular LH surges; low luteal progesterone; free T3 low, reverse T3 ↑
- *Risks:* Early ovulatory disruption, disordered eating/underfueling leads to vitamin deficiencies, stress fracture risk

30s: Adrenals and Ovaries Under Strain

- *Symptoms:* Infertility, implantation failure, heavy or anovulatory bleeding, fatigue, OCD tendencies, depression
- *Labs reveal:* Flattened cortisol curve, DHEA ↓; low luteal progesterone, estradiol suboptimal; free T3 low, reverse T3 ↑
- *Risks:* Subclinical hypothyroidism, amenorrhea, estrogen deficiency, diminished ovarian reserve, insulin resistance, postpartum depression/anxiety, immune dysregulation, injury risk

40s: Thyroid and Metabolic Fallout

- *Symptoms:* Hot flashes, brain fog, stubborn weight, IBS-like gut issues
- *Labs reveal:* AMH ↓, FSH ↑; thyroid labs suboptimal (TSH creeping up, free T3 low); hs-CRP ↑, A1c trending ↑
- *Risks:* Early or difficult perimenopause, osteoporosis/osteopenia, metabolic syndrome, autoimmunity

Symptoms Become Conditions

Unless something changes, the trajectory for an Achiever can shift from "competitor who loves winning" to "crumbling apart from over-exerting for so long."

When left unattended, over time:

- Brain-driven GnRH suppression can lead to functional hypothalamic amenorrhea, infertility, and recurrent implantation failure.

- Adrenal and ovarian strain becomes a luteal phase defect, low progesterone, early perimenopausal symptoms, and gut issues.
- Thyroid and metabolic slowdown can lead to hypothyroid patterns, weight dysregulation, and fatigue.

Whether the negative cascade has been happening for months, years, or decades, it is never too late to change the direction of the snowball. I have treated extremely burnt-out, depleted Achievers in their 40s and even 50s who create remarkable shifts that we can see in their follow-up lab testing and that they can *feel*. The path to healing begins by adopting this belief: "It's not too late."

The Flourishing Achiever

When the Achiever reaches a 10 on the Wellness Spectrum, she is unstoppable. She is still ambitious and driven. That hasn't changed. But now, she moves at a humane and sustainable pace. Think: an elite athlete who is well-rested and well-fueled, rather than one who is running on empty. Now she is more powerful than ever.

Before, she used to push to extremes. Now, she appreciates the beauty of taking a more moderate path. She now believes, "Rest is fuel, not laziness." "Taking time to recharge is essential." "Extreme measures don't get me where I want to be; a more moderate and/or efficient, sustainable path does." "I can be all the things I want to be, successful, accomplished, a winner, without pushing myself so brutally hard."

What the Achiever Needs Most

How can the Achiever reach a 10 on the Wellness Spectrum?

If you're an Achiever, your primary assignment is to find ways to rest and refuel. If you want to perform at an elite level, then you can't be running on fumes.

What are some ways to rest and refuel? As an Achiever, this might look like:

- Reducing the number of high-intensity workouts you do in each week and adding gentler forms of movement to your routine or highly efficient strength training.
- Building more recovery time in your routine so that you can recover after a big athletic event or after an especially busy season at work.
- Downshifting your work schedule from 50+ hours a week to 40, 30, or 20 hours. Or taking screen-free days to unplug completely from work.
- Practicing slow-motion time. A slow walk. Slow stretching. Enjoying a slow and unhurried conversation. Slowing down is powerful medicine for the Achiever.
- Reconnecting with the parts of your identity and life that have nothing to do with "achievement." Such as leisure, travel, play, creativity, and friendship, purely for the joy of it.

Resting does not always mean "sleeping." Rest is anything that replenishes you, rather than placing greater demands on your body and mind.

Slowing down and focusing on restorative activities can feel very uncomfortable. Remember, as an Achiever, your nervous system perceives safety when you feel successful. You may think, "If I slow down, then I won't be as successful," and this can feel threatening to your sensitive nervous system. Even if you recognize logically that being gentler with yourself is a good idea, your nervous system's primal wiring may not agree. Therefore, although you know you ought to make specific changes, you resist doing it because your highest, wisest self is locked in a disagreement with your nervous system.

What you need to do is retrain your nervous system to perceive safety in a new way. This looks like gradually training yourself to believe, "I can slow down and still achieve many of my goals," "I can feel good about myself even if I don't achieve certain goals." Eventually, "I am safe even if I achieve *nothing* today," or "Achievement involves deep rest combined with efficient training/work so that I can reach my highest potential."

How do you build these new beliefs, which may seem so foreign right now? By gathering tiny pieces of evidence that confirm these beliefs are true. For instance, when you choose to end your workday at 4 p.m. rather than 8 p.m. and still have a productive day, consider this another coin in your evidence bank. This is proof that you don't have to push so hard to achieve what you desire. As the evidence stacks up, your mindset softens, your beliefs evolve, and your stubborn nervous system begins to shift.

Achiever, your assignment is to rest, seek moderation, and pursue balance, not extremes. Remember that the very thing you are resisting is the very thing you need most.

If your Hormone Type is the Achiever, **how can you rest and refuel today?**

Key Takeaways

- The Achiever tends to be highly competitive. Whether in athletics, a corporate career, or anything else, she loves to push herself to extremes and win first place.
- Pushing so hard, without taking adequate time to rest and refuel, takes a toll on the Achiever's hormonal well-being.
- Over time, her brain (particularly the hypothalamus and pituitary glands) suffers under the strain. Later, her adrenals and ovaries are impacted. Finally, her thyroid and metabolic health become impaired.
- When out of balance, the most common emotional symptoms for an Achiever are volatile self-esteem (when she's winning, she feels great about herself, but that feeling rarely lasts), perfectionism, and a heightened need for control.

- The most common cognitive symptoms are rigid and inflexible thinking, depressive symptoms, intrusive thoughts, OCD-like traits, and negative attitudes about food and body image, which lead to disordered eating.
- Common physical symptoms include irregular or absent menstrual periods and gonadal insufficiency. Decreased uterine, skin, and brain health; low libido; bone loss (osteoporosis/osteopenia); hot flashes; and premature aging are all hallmark signs of an Achiever in distress.
- To turn the negative hormonal snowball into a positive one, the Achiever's assignment is to build rest and recovery into her routine.
- At first, slowing down can be unsettling for the Achiever and feel threatening to her nervous system. But over time, her nervous system can be rewired to this new reality.
- A well-rested Achiever is an unstoppable force. Rest allows her to do more, not less.

Notes

1. "A Systematic Review of Misdiagnosis in Those with Obsessive-Compulsive Disorder." Science Direct. Brittany Stahnke. 2021. https://www.sciencedirect.com/science/article/pii/S2666915321001578.
2. "Menstruation in Girls and Adolescents: Using the Menstrual Cycle as a Vital Sign." Obstetrics & Gynecology. Committee on Adolescent Health Care, American College of Obstetricians and Gynecologists. 2015. https://www.acog.org/clinical/clinical-guidance/committee-opinion/articles/2015/12/menstruation-in-girls-and-adolescents-using-the-menstrual-cycle-as-a-vital-sigis ton.

Chapter 5

The Survivor

Linda is in her 50s but appears a decade older. Meeting with her for the first time, I notice that she's carrying some extra weight on her body, her shoulders cave forward slightly, and her upper back is rounded. It brings to mind the image of a turtle shell. Energetically, it's as though her body has constructed a shield around itself, a protective layering, so that nothing can pierce through.

Over several appointments, she tells me bits and pieces of her story, and I begin to see the bigger picture.

This woman has been through a *lot*. A difficult childhood. A complicated marriage that ended painfully when she discovered her husband's infidelity. To top it all off, she was handed challenging genetics, including a family predisposition toward cancer. Linda already battled cancer once and got through it, but the invasive treatments took a tremendous toll on her body.

She describes her symptoms, digestive issues, constipation, and excess weight she can't seem to lose. A mysterious cyst that keeps growing back. Brain fog that never seems to lift. Ongoing sinus congestion with no apparent cause, and she wonders if it's due to allergies, mold, or something else.

As our conversations continue, she explains that she has felt stuck for a long time. Not just physically, but emotionally too. She hasn't dated anyone since the divorce, which was more than a decade ago, and the idea of opening herself up to potential rejection and heartache sounds incredibly unappealing. *No thanks*. Her home is her comfort zone, where she can zone out with a Netflix show and where she feels secure and safe. One of her kids is in college in another state, the other still lives at home but will be moving out soon, and she feels a mix of complicated emotions about becoming an empty nester. While her ex-husband, her kids, and others around her seem to be moving onward and upward with their lives, she feels stagnant.

Linda hasn't felt vibrant or beautiful in a long time and wonders if she ever will again. She is beginning to lose hope that change is possible.

Seeing Linda, some might think, "She looks defeated," or "There's a woman who has really let herself go and who has given up on life." But that's not what I see.

I see a Survivor.

Out of all the Hormone Types—Caretaker, Achiever, and Survivor—my Survivor patients are the ones who tend to be the most stuck but, also, who experience the most dramatic and exciting transformations.

How the Survivor Presents

When hormonally out of balance, Survivors emanate a stagnant, clogged energy. This type often has challenging genetic coding, such as a genetic predisposition toward cancer, diabetes, depression, and other conditions. In addition, the Survivor is a woman who has often endured a great deal of pain due to abandonment, abuse, divorce, discrimination, a chronic illness, and other difficult experiences. She carries a heavy load, physically and emotionally.

The combination of genetic challenges plus challenging life circumstances overloads the various systems in her body, making her more vulnerable to environmental toxins and allergens than other types.

Imagine a pipe already halfway clogged and then pouring a thick goo into it. Now it's completely stuffed up. Because Survivors are already at a disadvantage, health-wise, things like mold, mildew, or pollen that another woman might tolerate can wreak havoc on a Survivor. Her body says, "I'm already handling more than I can manage. I can't take on this, too."

The Survivor can present as:

Someone with a **chronic illness** that persists, with little to no improvement, leading to hopeless feelings	A woman who feels **stagnant and stuck** in her career, stuck in a relationship that's not working, stuck financially, or immobilized in another way	Someone who has been through difficult events and who is struggling to release the **pain of the past**

Caretakers, Achievers, and Survivors all have the capacity to become stuck in unhealthy patterns. But out of the three types, Survivors are the ones who tend to get deeply entrenched and have the most difficulty dislodging. The longer the stuck feeling persists, without relief, the lower the Survivor sinks on the Wellness Spectrum.

The Wellness Spectrum

To refresh your memory, on the Wellness Spectrum, 0 indicates extreme distress and 10 indicates optimal health.

When I begin working with a Survivor, it can be tough to get them moving in the right direction, toward a 7, 8, 9, and eventually 10 on the Wellness Spectrum. Like a boulder stuck in the mud, the Survivor sometimes struggles to make changes. But to paraphrase Newton's First Law of Motion, an object at rest will stay at rest, and an object in motion will stay in motion. Once the Survivor starts moving, they are like a boulder gathering speed as it rolls down a mountain slope. Survivors can build *huge* momentum.

Some of the most extraordinary changes I have ever witnessed in my practice, dramatic body composition changes, mood changes, career changes, relationship changes, and complete life transformations, have been my Survivor patients.

You Might Be a Survivor If. . .

- You have dealt (or are currently dealing with) considerable pain or trauma in your life. There is a heaviness that you carry, energetically, that you want to release.
- Your ancestors were survivors (war, famine, poverty, disease, discrimination), and this is imprinted in your genetic coding. Your body remembers what it endured, even if you didn't personally experience it.
- You might have more genetic hurdles compared to other people, such as a genetic predisposition to weight gain or depression.
- You are especially sensitive to environmental issues (mold, mildew, allergens) and toxins (more sensitive than others). Because your system is already overburdened, external toxins push you over the edge.
- You have a misunderstood health condition that causes you distress, but others don't see it or don't believe it's real. You suffer in isolation and wish others understood.
- You struggle with a lethargic, clogged, stuck, or stagnant sensation emotionally, physically, or both. This can manifest as constipation, weight gain, a chronically stuffed nose, or feeling depressed, blue, or unmotivated.
- You often have difficulty getting into a "flow" and "getting moving" with specific goals or projects.

The Survivor's Most Common Symptoms

Unpleasant symptoms are like a text message alert from your body, letting you know, "Hey, something is off and needs your attention." When the Survivor is at a 9 or 10 on the Wellness Spectrum, in a state of optimal health, she will have few or no symptoms, or very mild ones. But when she sinks to a lower number, these are the most common symptoms that appear. Not all Survivors experience these symptoms, but many do.

Emotional Symptoms

Low or depressed mood: Depression is common for Survivors. Some of my Survivor patients meet the clinical criteria for a depressive mood disorder, and some don't. A low, blue, or hopeless mood is very prevalent.

Wondering if you meet the criteria for clinical depression? There are several validated self-assessment tools you can use, including the Patient Health Questionnaire-9 (PHQ-9), the Beck Depression Inventory (BDI), and the Depression, Anxiety, and Stress Scale (DASS-21). Search online to find these assessments available for free.

If you have a newborn or infant and wonder if you may have postpartum depression, the Edinburgh Postnatal Depression Scale (EPDS) is a widely used assessment. These assessments ask a series of questions about your mood, energy levels, appetite, and other topics, and your score indicates if you may be experiencing depression and, if so, to what degree of severity.

Although everyone feels down from time to time, depression is more than just feeling "a bit low," because it can impair your quality of life and ability to function.

Whether you meet the clinical criteria or not, if you are experiencing persistent feelings of sadness, apathy, loss of interest in things you used to enjoy or care about, or feel hopeless about the future, especially if these feelings last for more than two weeks,[1] *it is vital to seek help from a therapist or another qualified provider.*

A note on antidepressants and hormones: as you're learning throughout this book, hormonal imbalances can lead to depression and amplify symptoms. This is why, for many women

I treat, taking an antidepressant may be given as a temporary solution (especially for those who are more severely impacted). Still, it is not a complete solution.

While antidepressants can be the right choice for some, these medications don't address the underlying hormonal imbalances and can even worsen hormonal dysregulation if the underlying concerns go unaddressed. Some antidepressants have been shown to impact estrogen levels, though this can vary from woman to woman, as every individual responds differently to meds.[2] The bottom line: while antidepressants may help with some symptoms of depression, for most, it is not a complete solution. The underlying hormonal issues remain. This is why I always recommend a wellness plan that centers on restoring hormonal health, not an afterthought.

Feeling stuck: Many Survivors want their health and lives to change but struggle to motivate themselves to take action consistently. Unlike the Caretaker, who tends to keep herself extremely busy, and the Achiever, who is proactive and goal-oriented, the Survivor is more likely to feel stuck. The Survivor might feel tremendous resistance to change, self-sabotage, and take actions that lead in the opposite direction, and struggle to get (and stay) moving.

Cognitive Symptoms

Brain fog and memory issues: Due to their tendency toward depression, many Survivors experience brain fog. This can manifest as slower processing speed, difficulty with planning and problem-solving, having a harder time learning new skills, or retaining new information.

Memory issues are common for Survivors. This is partly because depression can cause changes in brain structure and function. Research shows that the hippocampus (the part of your brain that plays a role in memory, spatial navigation, and emotional responses) can shrink in individuals with depression. Depression can also impair the prefrontal cortex, the region of the brain that controls decision-making, focus, and planning.[3]

For my Survivor patients, this can translate into difficulty making decisions or acting on ideas and a hazy feeling in their minds, like it's hard to think clearly or move forward with plans. This contributes to the "stuck" feeling that many Survivors report.

Physical Symptoms

Slow metabolism: Survivors often experience a slowed or sluggish metabolism. This can manifest as weight gain, especially around the midsection, despite unchanged food intake. Research[4] shows[5] that chronic stress and trauma dysregulate the hypothalamic-pituitary-adrenal (HPA) axis, leading to higher cortisol exposure, insulin resistance, and a "metabolic brake" that makes weight release especially challenging. Many Survivors describe feeling like their body is "holding on" despite healthy changes in diet or movement.

Gut and liver dysregulation: Digestive complaints are almost universal in this type. Bloating, constipation, reflux, and abdominal discomfort often show up, reflecting how unresolved trauma and chronic stress can alter the gut microbiome, slow motility, and compromise digestion.[6] The liver, overburdened with environmental toxins, past medications (like chemotherapy or long-term pharmaceuticals), and hormone metabolites, may also struggle to keep pace. This can present as poor detox capacity—sensitivity to alcohol, caffeine, medications, or even chemical smells. Some Survivors also develop recurring cysts or growths, reflecting stagnant detox and elimination pathways.

Fatigue/low energy: Persistent fatigue is another hallmark symptom when a Survivor is hormonally out of whack. Even with adequate sleep, Survivors may feel unrefreshed, sluggish, or weighed down by exhaustion. This stems from mitochondrial dysfunction and reduced energy production at the cellular level, often seen after chronic stress, trauma, or repeated illness. It's not just tiredness; it's the sense that your body is moving through quicksand.

Over time, this fatigue seeps into the Survivor's mood, motivation, and the ability to engage fully in life.

Nervous System Wiring: Safety and Threats for the Survivor

As a quick review of what we covered in previous chapters, your nervous system continually scans your environment, looking for potential threats. Messages travel through your brain, spinal cord, and a network of nerves throughout your body to say either "We're safe right now" or "We're not safe."

Your nervous system's job is to protect you from danger. However, the nervous system's focus on self-preservation can also be counterproductive.

Because of the trauma they have experienced, my Survivor patients tend to go overboard when it comes to creating a sense of safety. They might self-soothe with food, alcohol, cannabis, or by burrowing into environments that feel secure and protected. Think: the homebody who rarely goes out, preferring to stay home in her cocoon surrounded by creature comforts. These self-soothing measures protect the Survivor from experiencing further pain but also make her life smaller than it needs to be.

Some (though not all) Survivors develop a cynical outlook toward life, and their beliefs sound like this: "The odds are stacked against me." "The world is not a safe place." "People have abandoned me in the past and will again."

Others remain optimistic that change is possible, but over time, their optimism begins to dwindle. After repeated disappointments, she begins to believe, "I have been stuck for a long time, and it's unlikely to change." "I'm not sure I have what it takes to improve my life. I have tried before, but it hasn't worked out." "I don't want to try and be disappointed yet again."

In various ways, **the Survivor believes that the world is not a safe place and in response builds a protective wall around herself.** Shielding herself from people, places, or experiences that might provoke uncomfortable feelings, especially rejection, sadness, or disappointment.

What threatens the Survivor's sense of safety is removing the protective armor and allowing herself to hope and try again. For her, this feels vulnerable and scary. It is also the most powerful step she can take toward optimum health.

What the Survivor needs most of all is a willingness to keep trying again, to get moving, and to welcome fresh energy and new experiences into her life.

The Survivor		
Safety	**Threat**	**Shift**
She feels safe when she perceives: "I am in my cozy cocoon, shielded, protected. Nothing can hurt me here."	She feels unsafe when she perceives: "I am vulnerable to rejection, disappointment, or another form of pain."	She achieves optimal wellness when she shifts to a new set of beliefs: "I can remove my protective covering and still be safe." "It is safe to feel optimistic about the future, to allow myself to hope and trust again." "Even if I do experience disappointment or hurt, I am resilient and I can handle it."

What's Happening on a Biomedical Level

When the Survivor Is Not Well: First, Second, and Third Levels of Impact

When the Survivor's hormones are out of balance, it's her *gut health* that takes center stage. Her digestion, nutrient absorption, and the microbiome are the first to be impacted.

When working with my Survivor patients, I often see dysbiosis, low-diversity microbiota, slowed motility/constipation, and increased intestinal permeability (aka "leaky gut"), which raises the liver's antigen/toxin load via the portal vein–gut–liver axis.

The primary portal vein in the body is the hepatic portal vein, which carries blood from your digestive tract, gallbladder, pancreas, and spleen to the liver, where toxins get filtered out by your hard-working liver before the purified blood gets transported back to your heart. When a Survivor is unwell, bacterial products, especially lipopolysaccharide (LPS), can leak into the Survivor's portal blood, amplifying hepatic and systemic low-grade inflammation and insulin resistance, also known as metabolic endotoxemia. Gut health is the first to suffer. *Liver function* is the second level of impact, leading to impaired detoxification, hormone clearance, and bile metabolism.

Your liver's job is to clear xenobiotics (chemical substances such as pesticides, pollutants, and food additives), alcohol, medications, hormone metabolites, and microbial products from your blood, while also managing bile acid synthesis/recycling.

When overloaded with toxins, the liver can't keep up. Bile flow stagnates. The risk for steatosis or nonalcoholic fatty liver disease, aka MASLD/NAFLD, a condition where excess fat builds up in the liver, rises. The bile acids that regulate glucose, lipids, and glucagon-like peptide-1 (GLP-1), a hormone that helps regulate blood sugar and appetite, struggle to do their jobs, worsening metabolism even further.

As her gut and liver become strained, the domino effect continues, and the Survivor's *metabolic and mitochondrial health* are the third level of impact. This leads to issues with energy production, insulin sensitivity, and overall vitality.

Chronic inflammation and nutrient shortfalls impair the Survivor's mitochondrial ATP output (ATP is adenosine triphosphate, the energy-carrying molecule that powers your cells to function), raise oxidative stress, and blunt thyroid-driven energy metabolism. After doing lab testing for a Survivor, I often see less T3 action and more (rT3) reverse triiodothyronine, a metabolically inactive form of the thyroid hormone triiodothyronine (aka T3).

rT3 is a hormone that instructs your metabolism to slow down. If you are stranded on a deserted island and starving, you want rT3 because it helps your body slow its processes, conserve energy, and stay alive longer without fuel. But for day-to-day life? Too much rT3 is not helpful because it makes your metabolism slower than it ought to be. For the Survivor, trauma and chronic stress further deplete mitochondrial defenses and resilience. The result? Sluggish metabolism, fatigue, and weight gain.

Estrogen dysregulation is also common for my Survivor patients. This happens because the estrobolome (gut microbiomes that metabolize estrogen, also known as microbial β-glucuronidase) is overactive. This can raise recirculating estrogen, fueling estrogen-sensitive symptoms and growths (think: recurring cysts) or, conversely, contribute to estrogen depletion when microbiome diversity is low and bile flow is poor. See Figure 5.1.

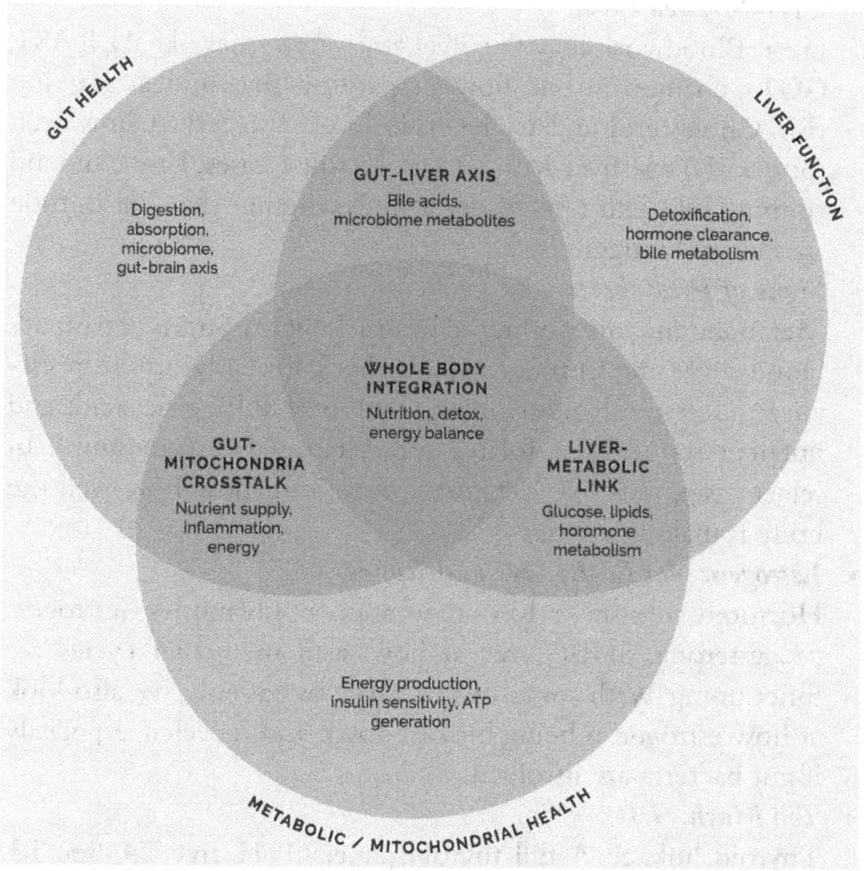

Figure 5.1 Gut health and interconnected systems.

What the Lab Testing Shows

When a Survivor comes into my clinic and describes her symptoms, constipation, weight gain, a feeling of stuckness and stagnation, to name a few, and we begin doing lab testing, this is what I typically find in her results:

- ***Low Diversity in Gut Bacteria***
  Gut: Testing may show reduced diversity of healthy bacteria, signs of inflammation, or an enzyme (β-glucuronidase) that allows estrogen to recirculate too much. Slow digestion can lead to methane-producing microbes. Unless there's a bigger problem, blood in the stool usually won't be present.
- ***Over-Stressed Liver***
  Liver: Bloodwork may flag liver stress (enzymes like ALT, AST, GGT), changes in bile flow, or patterns that hint at scarring risk. Cholesterol and triglyceride levels also reflect how well (or poorly) the liver handles fats. In some cases, I recommend running bile acid tests to determine whether they are outside the optimal ranges.
- ***Signs of Prediabetes***
  Metabolic and mitochondrial health: I test my Survivor patient's blood sugar and insulin levels to check for early insulin resistance; cholesterol ratios; inflammation (CRP); uric acid; and nutrient status (B12, folate, iron, vitamin D, magnesium). In select cases, tests like lactate/pyruvate can show how well the body is making energy.
- ***Estrogen: Not in the Optimal Range***
  Hormone crosstalk: Key reproductive hormones (estrogen, progesterone, SHBG) reveal how well menstrual cycles are functioning. With some of my Survivor patients, we also look at how estrogen is being broken down and recycled, especially if gut bacteria are involved.
- ***Too Much rT3***
  Thyroid linkage: A full thyroid panel (TSH, free T4, free T3, reverse T3) shows how well the liver converts thyroid hormones into their active forms. Thyroid antibodies can be checked if autoimmunity is suspected.

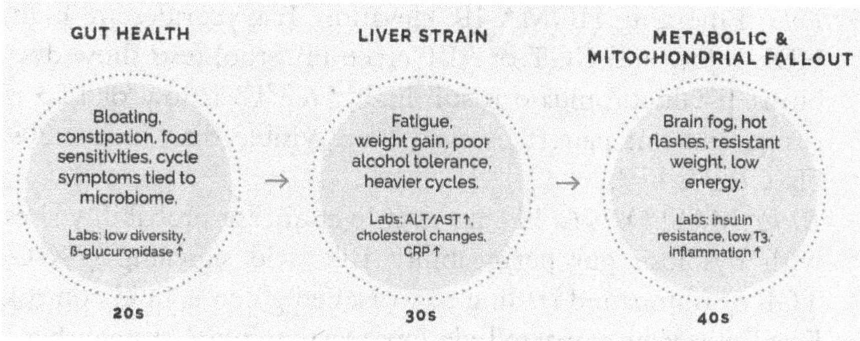

Figure 5.2 Progression across the decades: gut to liver to metabolic/mitochondrial.

Decade by Decade: How the Negative Snowball Rolls

If you're a Survivor, and your hormones are out of balance, here's how the negative snowball tends to build momentum through the decades (see Figure 5.2):

20s: Gut-First Hints

- *Symptoms:* Bloating, constipation, food sensitivities, acne, or PMS swings suggest estrogen imbalance. Weight fluctuation despite "clean eating."
- *Labs reveal:* Stool diversity is low. β-Glucuronidase is high (especially if there are estrogen recirculation issues). Ferritin and B12 are on the lower end of normal. ALT/AST are often normal, but hs-CRP can trend upward. Fasting insulin is borderline. Free T3 is also at the lower end of normal, with rT3 slightly high in high-stress/low-food intake periods.
- *Risks:* Early dysbiosis can lead to metabolic endotoxemia, which seeds insulin resistance. Estrogen-related symptoms (cyclical breast tenderness, heavier bleeds) if β-glucuronidase is high.[7]

30s: Liver Overload and Metabolic Creep

- *Symptoms:* Stubborn weight around the midsection. Fatigue that is not fixed by sleep. Heavier or more symptomatic menstrual cycles. Feeling burdened by toxins (many Survivors tell me, "I can't tolerate alcohol anymore"). Detox capacity feels reduced.

- *Labs:* Emerging HOMA-IR elevation. Triglycerides are high, HDL is low, and GGT or ALT creep up. Stool tests show dysbiosis. β-Glucuronidase is still high. Free T3 is low or rT3 is rising, and this pattern is even more visible than in her 20s. Hs-CRP is high.
- *Risks:* MASLD/NAFLD, aka fatty liver disease, probability rises with dysbiosis/gut permeability. Bile acid signaling (FXR/TGR5) is impaired leading to worsened glucose/lipid control. Fertility can be impacted via low progesterone/estrogen handling problems.[8]

40s: Mitochondrial and Systemic Fallout

- *Symptoms:* Low energy, brain fog, hot flashes, and night sweats hit harder. IBS-like symptoms persist. Weight resistant to change. Joint aches.
- *Labs:* A1c and fasting insulin are high, triglycerides are high, hs-CRP is high. DEXA may show early osteopenia if nutrition/estrogen has been suboptimal long-term. Liver ultrasound may show steatosis. Free T3 is low, rT3 is high despite TSH being in the upper-normal range. Stool diversity is low.
- *Risks:* Metabolic syndrome, progression of MASLD/NAFLD, gallbladder/bile flow issues, higher overall inflammatory tone that amplifies perimenopause symptoms.[9]

Symptoms Become Conditions

If left unmanaged, the trajectory for a Survivor can shift from feeling "low and stuck" to "severely unwell," with her gut, liver, and other organs and glands buckling under the strain.

Without intervention, over time:

- Dysbiosis and gut permeability lead to IBS phenotype, metabolic endotoxemia, insulin resistance, and, in some cases, MASLD/NAFLD.[10]
- Bile acid signaling failure can lead to impaired FXR/TGR5 signaling, worsening glucose and lipid regulation and dulling

GLP-1 responses. (This is part of the reason why so many Survivors struggle with stubborn weight gain.)

- Estrobolome imbalance becomes an estrogen recirculation pattern (this manifests as breast tenderness, excessive uterine thickening during cycles, and heavy bleeds) or, with severe dysbiosis and low bile flow, relative estrogen insufficiency symptoms such as hot flashes, night sweats, mood changes, and vaginal dryness.[11]
- Liver-thyroid coupling failure leads to a low-T3/high-rT3 pattern with fatigue, weight gain, cold intolerance, despite "normal" TSH levels because hepatic D1 conversion is impaired.[12]
- Chronic trauma/stress overload later shows up as mitochondrial vulnerability, oxidative stress, and slower cellular repair—amplifying depression and fatigue and blunting lifestyle response.[13,14]

Remember the woman I described at the start of this chapter? Linda's health history—early childhood trauma, cancer therapy, long-standing constipation, weight gain, chemical sensitivity, recurrent cysts, and cognitive slowing—tracks with the gut-first, liver-overloaded, metabolic, and mitochondrial-depleted pattern that is common with Survivors.

But women like Linda can make astounding changes. Even in your 50s and beyond, creating a massive turnaround is within reach.

The Flourishing Survivor

In optimal health, the Survivor is a powerful role model who embodies perseverance and triumph over the odds. Many influential writers, teachers, coaches, and speakers are Survivors who have found their way out of the dark and back into the light, and who use their stories to inspire others and spread a message of hope.

Survivors also have tremendous compassion for others, because they understand firsthand how difficult life can be. They extend patience and grace to others when they are struggling. I have found that, once they are feeling better, my Survivor patients often have incredible appreciation for the gift of life ("I am so grateful to be alive and feel good!") because they know what it's like on the other side of the spectrum and know how bad things can get.

What the Survivor Needs Most

How can the Survivor reach a 10 on the Wellness Spectrum?

If you're a Survivor type, your first assignment is to open the channels so that fresh energy can flow through you.

Get moving, literally and energetically. Get yourself out of the house. Take an invigorating walk. Spend time in nature or with a loved one. Sign up for a class and expose yourself to new people and ideas. Back at home, deep-clean your house, open the windows, and let in the light and fresh air. Bravely open yourself up to new experiences and new possibilities, even though this may feel emotionally risky.

I also recommend surrounding yourself with symbols of hope. Listen to podcasts or audiobooks about people who have made massive changes in their lives. Reinforce the belief that change is possible for you, too.

The more you infuse hope into your life and keep your energy moving, like a flowing river washing through you, the faster you will move toward flourishing health.

What happened to Linda? She shook up her routine and started volunteering a few times a month. She made some new friends, surrounding herself with positive, uplifting women who became her walking buddies and got her out of the house more often. She had her home treated for mold and mildew and ripped out the old carpeting that had been gradually acquiring grime for years. Emotionally and physically, she felt like she could breathe again. These changes didn't happen all at once. This was a gradual progression of decisions, one choice leading to the next, over the course of a year or so.

She's still in therapy to work through traumatic experiences from the past, but overall, she feels "happier than I have felt in a long time." There's a new sparkle in her eyes, a brightness and lightness in her spirit that others can sense. She feels it, too. The pipes have been cleared out. The Survivor is now thriving.

Survivor, fresh energy, and forward motion are the medicine you need. If your Hormone Type is the Survivor, **how can you get yourself moving today?**

Key Takeaways

- The Survivor often struggles with lethargy and a stuck, stagnant feeling.
- Often, she is a woman who has a genetic predisposition toward physical or mental health conditions (the genetic cards are not stacked in her favor), and, on top of this, she may have experienced trauma in her life.
- When the Survivor is hormonally out of sync, her gut is the first to suffer, followed by her liver, which then leads to metabolic and mitochondrial issues.
- When out of balance, the most common emotional symptoms for a Survivor are a low or depressed mood and feelings of stuckness and resistance (wanting to make changes but struggling to do so).
- The most common cognitive symptoms are brain fog, memory issues, difficulty with focus, decision-making, and planning.
- Common physical symptoms include slow metabolism, digestive issues, recurring cysts or growths, heavy periods due to excessive uterine lining build-up, and fatigue that doesn't improve even with adequate sleep.

- The Survivor has a tendency to put up protective shields to avoid feeling pain. Removing the armor and opening herself up to new experiences is what the Survivor needs. Fresh air can't flow into a home when the windows are closed.
- To turn the negative hormonal snowball into a positive one, the Survivor's primary assignment is to combat stagnation by creating movement in her life, physically, mentally, and emotionally.
- This can look like moving her body regularly, decluttering and detoxifying her home, or building new, positive relationships. Motion, in all forms, is the medicine she needs.
- Survivors often make wonderful healers, therapists, and spiritual counselors because of their understanding of what it means to suffer and their compassion and empathy for those who are struggling with challenges. They've been there and can offer wisdom to others.
- Of the three Hormone Types, Survivors are the ones who often experience the most dramatic changes. Significant weight loss. Major shift in mood. Like debris being cleared from a river, allowing water to flow freely, monumental change is possible for the Survivor once she has the proper support and plan.

Notes

1. "Clinical Depression (Major Depressive Disorder)." Cleveland Clinic. Cleveland Clinic. 2022. https://my.clevelandclinic.org/health/diseases/24481-clinical-depression-major-depressive-disorder.
2. "Side Effects of Antidepressants in Females – What Women Should Know." Lindner Center of HOPE. Danielle Johnson, MD. 2024. https://lindnercenterofhope.org/blog/side-effects-antidepressants-women/.

3. "Does Depression Cause Memory Loss?" TMS Institute of Arizona. TMS Institute. 2025. https://tmsinstitute.co/does-depression-cause-memory-loss/.
4. Lengton, R., et al. (2024). Glucocorticoids and HPA Axis Regulation in the Stress–Obesity Connection: A Comprehensive Overview of Biological, Physiological and Behavioural Dimensions. *Clinical Obesity*. https://onlinelibrary.wiley.com/doi/10.1111/cob.12725.
5. Murphy, M., et al. (2022). Childhood Trauma, the HPA Axis and Psychiatric Illnesses: A Targeted Literature Synthesis. *Frontiers in Psychiatry*. https://www.frontiersin.org/journals/psychiatry/articles/10.3389/fpsyt.2022.748372/full.
6. Kelly, L. S., et al. (2021). Stress-Related Changes in the Gut Microbiome After Trauma. *Journal of Trauma and Acute Care Surgery*. https://journals.lww.com/jtrauma/abstract/2021/07000/stress_related_changes_in_the_gut_microbiome_after.28.aspx.
7. Boutagy, N. E., et al. (2016). Metabolic Endotoxemia with Obesity: Is It Real and Is It Relevant? https://pubmed.ncbi.nlm.nih.gov/26133659/.
8. Song, Q., & Zhang, X. (2022). The Role of Gut–Liver Axis in Gut Microbiome Dysbiosis Associated NAFLD and NAFLD-HCC. *Biomedicines*. https://pubmed.ncbi.nlm.nih.gov/35327326/.
9. Pezzino, S., et al. (2022). Gut-Liver Axis and Non-Alcoholic Fatty Liver Disease: A Vicious Circle of Dysfunctions Orchestrated by the Gut Microbiome. *Biology (Basel)*. https://pubmed.ncbi.nlm.nih.gov/36358323/.
10. Cani, P. D., et al. (2007). Metabolic endotoxemia initiates obesity and insulin resistance. *Diabetes*. https://pubmed.ncbi.nlm.nih.gov/17456850/.
11. Ervin, S. M., et al. (2019). Gut Microbial β-glucuronidases Reactivate Estrogens as Components of the Estrobolome. *Journal of Biological Chemistry*. https://pmc.ncbi.nlm.nih.gov/articles/PMC6901331/.

12. Bruinstroop, E., et al. (2023). Role of Hepatic Deiodinases in Thyroid Hormone Homeostasis and Liver Metabolism, Inflammation, and Fibrosis. *European Thyroid Journal*. https://pubmed.ncbi.nlm.nih.gov/36892852/.
13. Bruinstroop, E., et al. (2023). Role of Hepatic Deiodinases in Thyroid Hormone Homeostasis and Liver Metabolism, Inflammation, and Fibrosis. *European Thyroid Journal*. https://pubmed.ncbi.nlm.nih.gov/36892852/.
14. Picard, M., et al. (2018). Mitochondrial Dysfunction and Stress-Related Disorders. *Nature Reviews Neuroscience*. https://doi.org/10.1038/s41594-026-01769-9; and Epel, E.S., et al. (2018). Psychological Stress, Mitochondria, and Cellular Aging. *Nature Reviews Endocrinology*. https://doi.org/10.1016/j.arr.2023.10.145.

Part Three

CREATE YOUR HORMONE ACTION PLAN

Throughout this book, I have invited you to imagine wellness as a spectrum from 0–10. What score would you give yourself right now? For many of my clients, the answer is "maybe somewhere around a 5, not awful, but not great either," or "somewhere in the range of 3–7, depending on the day."

Wherever you are, my goal is to help you move closer to 10.

Now that we have reached *Part Three: Create Your Hormone Action Plan*, I'll take you through the action steps to get there.

The Seven Components of Your Hormone Action Plan

At my women's health clinic, the clients who achieve the best results: hormone levels coming back to the optimal ranges, mood lifting, energy rising, improved body composition, regular cycles, increased libido and fertility, all the positive signs we are hoping to see, are the ones who create a seven-part wellness plan (see Figure 6.1).

As you can see, "create your support network" is right at the center of the plan. Your support network may include family members who want you to thrive, friends who inspire you to take excellent care of yourself, service providers on your healthcare team, an online community of women or another group you are part of, and more. Once you have a strong support network in place, the other six pieces of your Hormone Action Plan become so much easier to do.

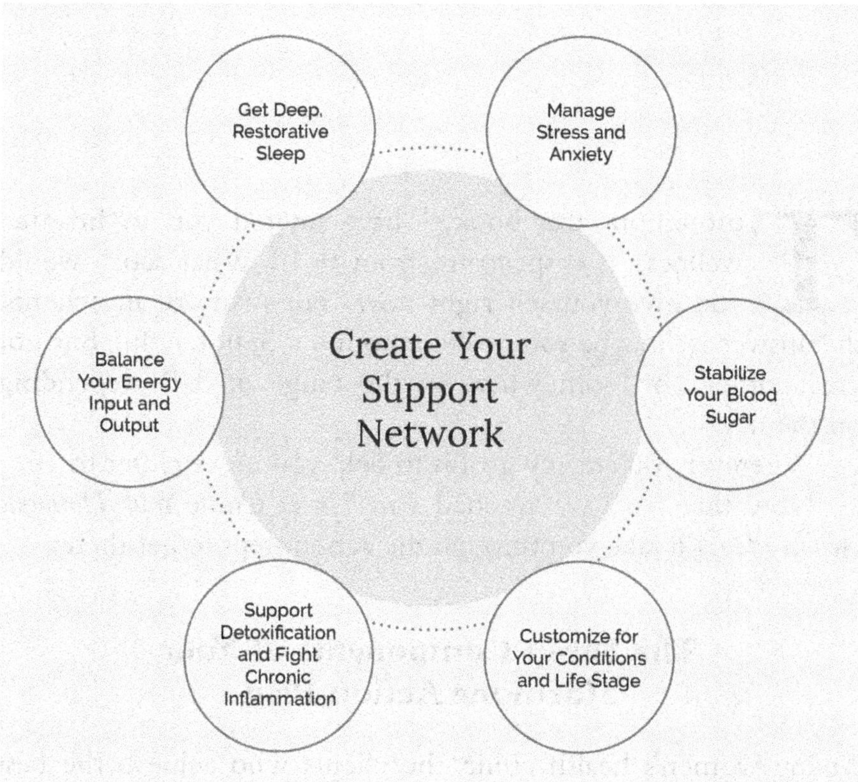

Figure 6.1 Your hormone action plan: the seven components

In Part Three, you'll find one chapter dedicated to each part of the plan, a chapter on how to manage stress and anxiety, one on how to stabilize your blood sugar, and so on. At the end of each chapter, I give a specific prescription for each hormone type. This is important because the prescription I recommend to a Caretaker might be different from the approach I'd recommend for an Achiever or Survivor. Personalizing the plan to your type is what leads to faster relief and lasting transformation.

Bringing It All Together

At the end of Part Three, I provide three sample Hormone Action Plans, one for each Hormone Type. While your personal plan may look a bit different, these sample plans show how all the details come together to form an action plan. I hope each sample plan inspires you to create your own!

The Therapeutic Order

Naturopathic doctors (NDs), like me, follow a set of guidelines called the *Therapeutic Order of Naturopathic Medicine*.[1] This guideline explains what NDs do with their patients and the order in which they do so. The Therapeutic Order is based on the idea that your body knows how to heal itself, and when given the proper support, it will. It consists of the following steps:

1. Establish the foundation for optimal health.
2. Stimulate self-healing.
3. Support and restore weakened systems.
4. Address physical alignments.
5. Natural symptom relief.
6. Synthetic symptom relief.
7. High force interventions.

The first phase of the Therapeutic Order is to "establish the foundation for optimal health." This means helping the patient to make healthy lifestyle shifts, creating a plan that will move her closer to a 10 on the Wellness Spectrum. The last phase is "high-force interventions," such as pharmaceutical drugs, surgery, chemotherapy, and other aggressive forms of treatment that can inflict lasting harm on the body. Naturopathic doctors focus on the least invasive options first, escalating to more invasive options later and only if needed.

To quote the Association of Accredited Naturopathic Medical Colleges, the purpose of the Therapeutic Order is to "use the least amount of force [...] to promote gentle, safe and long-lasting health and well-being" in order "to maximize patient benefit and reduce the potential for damage or harm."[2]

Your Hormone Action Plan is guided by this Therapeutic Order. We begin with the options that help the most, while inflicting the least harm. If, after implementing your plan, you are still not seeing the results you hoped for, you can talk to your ND or another provider about the higher levels of the order, synthetic symptom relief or high-force interventions, and discuss whether these are right for you.

One Choice, Many Benefits

Most of my patients are busy women who carry *a lot*. The thought of adding even just "one more thing" to their already stuffed to-do list feels overwhelming. You may be feeling the same way and thinking, "Yes, I want to feel better. I want to be the healthiest, most flourishing version of me. . .but how am I supposed to incorporate a seven-part wellness plan into my life?! There is just no space. . .."

I want to leave you with these words of reassurance.

Many parts of your Hormone Action Plan overlap and feed into one another. Just as all the hormonal communication highways in your body are connected, every piece of your wellness plan is, too.

Imagine that today you decide to take a short walk in the fresh air to a nearby cafe where you're meeting a friend for a nutritious, protein, and fiber-rich lunch. This one choice supports every single part of your Hormone Action Plan. You're managing stress and anxiety, stabilizing your blood sugar, setting yourself up for a night of deep sleep, moving and fueling your body for optimal hormonal balance, decreasing inflammation, healing chronic conditions, and strengthening your support network. With one action, you're checking off every single box in your plan.

So, rolling out your seven-part plan doesn't necessarily mean you're adding seven extra items to your daily to-do list! Often it means elevating the choices you're already making and choosing higher-quality, hormone-regulating options. It's about upgrading your routine, rather than adding "more" to it.

One small choice can support your hormonal health on many levels. And when you make positive choices repeatedly, they build and compound. Soon, the negative snowball all reverses direction. Instead of sinking to a 4, 3, or 2 on the Wellness Spectrum, you start spiraling upward toward a 7, 8, 9, and eventually a 10. I see this happen in my clinic every week. I know it is possible for you, too. Let's create your plan to get there!

Notes

1. "The Therapeutic Order." Association of Accredited Naturopathic Medical Colleges (AANMC). AANMC. 2019. https://aanmc.org/featured-articles/therapeutic-order/.
2. "The Therapeutic Order." Association of Accredited Naturopathic Medical Colleges (AANMC). AANMC. 2019. https://aanmc.org/featured-articles/therapeutic-order/.

Chapter 6

Manage Stress and Anxiety

There have been more mornings than I'd like to admit when I wake up already buzzing with anxiety. Before my feet even touch the floor, my mind is running: kids' lunches, patient calls, business deadlines, unread texts, a thousand small decisions waiting for me.

My heart races. My breath is shallow. And I think, I haven't even had tea yet—why does it feel like I'm already sprinting? If you've felt that too, you are not broken. You are living in a culture that keeps your nervous system on high alert. That's why we're tackling this first in your Hormone Action Plan. Because until stress is addressed, your hormones are always playing defense.

The Hormonal Cost of Chronic Stress

Stress activates your hypothalamic-pituitary-adrenal (HPA) axis—the communication highway between your brain and adrenal glands.

In an emergency, cortisol is brilliant. It sharpens focus, mobilizes glucose, increases blood flow, and gives you the surge you need to act quickly. You want cortisol when a toddler is about to fall or when something truly threatens your safety.

But when your cortisol levels stay high, all day, every day, it stops being protective and starts acting like a hormone thief. Your body reallocates resources to survival. Reproductive hormone signaling downshifts. Thyroid conversion slows. Blood sugar destabilizes. Sleep fragments. Over time, this shows up as irregular cycles, PMS, fertility challenges, central weight gain, anxiety, and exhaustion that no amount of coffee fixes.

The science runs deep.[1,2,3,4,5,6,7] Stress does not just "make you feel anxious." It reshapes endocrine communication, especially during life transitions, such as puberty, postpartum, and perimenopause, when hormones naturally fluctuate. It increases vulnerability to anxiety and depression, disrupts brain plasticity, and can even alter gene expression in ways that prime the brain for future mental health challenges.

Across decades, this matters. Chronic stress can suppress ovulation in your 20s, amplify PMS in your 30s, intensify perimenopausal symptoms in your 40s, challenge your fertility across all reproductive decades, and accelerate metabolic and bone changes later in life.

Simply put, unregulated stress taxes every hormonal system you rely on for vitality. However, when it comes to stress, there are nuances that many don't know about.

One of the most important nuances to understand? It's the fact that. . .

Not All Stress Is Bad

Stress isn't always the enemy. In fact, some stress is vital for gro wth.[8,9,10,11,12]

There's **distress**—the kind that keeps you awake at night, chips away at your vitality, and leaves you feeling depleted. Think: toxic work environments, unresolved trauma that haunts you, a brutal work schedule that's like a never-ending treadmill, or the relentless mental load of caregiving without support. This is the bad kind of stress that, when left unmanaged, can wreak havoc on your hormones.

But there's also **eustress**—the healthy kind of stress that challenges your system just enough to make it stronger. Eustress (from the ancient Greek word *eû*, which means "well" or "good") is a term coined by endocrinologist Hans Selye. Examples? Lifting weights or training for a race. Getting into a hot sauna or plunging into cold water. Tackling a big project you're passionate about. Taking a class that pushes you to think differently. All of these can be good forms of stress.

These are what my colleagues and I in the medical community refer to as **hormetic stressors**: small, intentional doses of stress that build resilience. Even fighting off a short-term fever can be considered a hormetic stressor, because placing your immune system under stress from a virus causes it to develop antibodies, making you less likely to get sick from the same bug again in the future.

Distress or Eustress?

How can you tell whether something is distress or eustress? In an article for the mental health website *Calmerry*, Kate Skurat, a writer with an MD in health and medical psychology, explains that distress[13] is marked by the following characteristics:

- Long-term
- Demotivating and exhausting
- Impairs your daily functioning
- Bigger than the resources you have to cope with it

Eustress, on the other hand, is stress that is:

- Short-term
- Motivating and energizing
- Allows you to build new tools
- And, you have adequate resources to handle it

When you are experiencing distress for a prolonged period—months, years, even decades—this is known as **chronic stress**. This is the kind of stress that takes the greatest toll on your body, because it's unrelenting, with no time to rest and recover.

What about **anxiety**? Think of anxiety as a stress multiplier. When you're experiencing distress, anxiety (spinning thoughts, worrying about future threats, or replaying past events in your mind) can make the stress feel even worse than it is. Stress burdens your body. Anxiety makes the load even heavier.

Reflect

What is one form of *distress* in your life?
Example: You are caring for your five-year-old and three-year-old, and working full time, with no village supporting you, and you are bone-crushingly exhausted.

What is one form of *eustress* in your life?
Example: You are training for a 5K race. The 10-week training process is physically and mentally demanding, but also exciting and energizing!

Meet Your Nervous System

Your nervous system has one primary question it asks all day:

Am I safe?

It does not differentiate well between a physical threat and an emotional one. A sharp email from your boss can trigger the same biochemical cascade as a near-miss car accident. Adrenaline rises. Cortisol follows. Blood sugar shifts. Heart rate increases.

Occasionally, this is adaptive. Chronically, it is exhausting.

When your body spends too much time in fight-or-flight mode, reproductive hormone signaling becomes secondary. Survival takes priority over ovulation, libido, and metabolic efficiency.

This is why managing stress is not a luxury. It is foundational hormone medicine.

> **A Note to Your Nervous System**
>
> Your nervous system is working hard to point out threats and keep you safe. But maybe it has been working a little *too* hard. If you could send an email or text to your nervous system, what would you say?
>
> Your message might be something like this:
>
> *Hi, nervous system, I appreciate that you're trying to point out potential threats and keep me safe. But we're going to start working together differently, because I don't need so many stress hormones flooding my body, so much of the time.*

What Does It Mean to Manage Stress and Anxiety?

When someone says, "It's important to learn how to manage your stress and anxiety," you may think, "Sure, sounds good, I totally agree. . .but what does this mean? Should I try to avoid stressful situations? Take more deep breaths? How do I actually do this?"

First, let's clarify that "manage" does not mean "eliminate." Your job is not to eliminate stress. It is to increase recovery and discern which stress is building you versus breaking you.

Managing stress does not mean pretending everything is fine. It does not mean avoiding responsibility. It does not mean becoming a monk on a mountain. It means building nervous system capacity.

Capacity is your ability to experience activation without losing your center and to return to baseline quickly when you are disrupted.

And this is where the *Top 5 Levers to Manage Stress Effectively* comes in.

Top 5 Levers to Manage Stress Effectively

1. Do daily nervous system hygiene.
2. Prioritize deep, restorative sleep.
3. Eat food that supports stress management.
4. Use botanical medicine helpers.
5. Do lab testing to check your stress hormone levels.

Do Daily Nervous System Hygiene

Dr. Niki Elliott, director of the Center for Embodied Equity and Neurodiversity at the University of San Diego, teaches people in high-burnout professions—like teachers, social workers, and administrators of foster care programs—how to manage their nervous systems more consciously to avoid burn out. Elliott uses the phrase "nervous system hygiene" to describe how this works. As she sums it up, every day, you brush your teeth without thinking about it. It's automatic. You just do it. Daily dental hygiene keeps your teeth strong and healthy and keeps your breath minty fresh. We never say we don't have time for it.

"Just like you practice dental hygiene every day," says Elliott, "You need to commit to practicing nervous system hygiene every day, too. Otherwise, your energy is off, and it definitely affects how you show up in service to others."

What are some ways to practice good nervous system hygiene? Pick one or more of the following options—all of which are evidence-based. Research on stress management confirms that these options really *do* work. These are some of the highest leverage moves you can make.

It doesn't matter which option you choose, as long as it's something you enjoy and can commit to doing regularly.

Nervous System Hygiene Options

- Do diaphragmatic breathing: find a quiet spot to sit or lie down. Place one hand on your chest and the other on your belly. Close your eyes, inhale slowly through your nose, and feel your belly expand. Exhale slowly through your mouth, and feel your belly slowly sink back down. Allow your exhale to be longer than the inhale. Repeat for a few minutes (ideally, 5 minutes).[14]
- Listen to music that promotes a settled nervous system.[15] Choose calming music that you love. Like breathing, this is one of the simplest ways to increase parasympathetic nervous system activity and decrease sympathetic overdrive. It's free and something you can do any time of day.
- Move your body in a way that feels good for you. Gentle movement like tai chi, stretching, or walking is a great option. But strength/resistance training can discharge stress and tension, too. Resistance training induces neural adaptations that enhance nervous system function, supporting both motor performance and cognitive health.[16] The key is that you're moving with intention, not to "burn calories" or to "punish yourself for what you ate earlier" but to signal safety to your body.
- Spend time in nature.[17] If that is not feasible, look at images of nature, or listen to a recording of nature sounds.

(continued)

(continued)

- Enjoy a few minutes engaged in a passion or hobby that brings you joy.[18]
- Do repetitive, rhythmic movement, like dancing, playing music, chopping vegetables, rolling dough, organizing clothes, coloring, or knitting.[19]
- Try acupuncture, acupressure, or emotional freedom technique (EFT),[20] which involves lightly tapping your fingers on various points on your body while reciting an empowering affirmation to yourself.
- Get a massage.[21]
- Listen to a guided relaxation meditation or visualization.[22]
- Connect with others, such as sharing what you're feeling honestly with a trusted friend, partner, or professional.
- Try a mindfulness-based therapy session, such as mindfulness-based cognitive therapy (MBCT), mindfulness-based stress reduction (MBSR), or dialectal behavior therapy (DBT).[23]
- Hold boundaries and say "no" to one more thing on your plate.

Why is it so important to do nervous system hygiene, daily? The benefits are twofold: one, to settle your nervous system when you feel agitated, and two, to increase your nervous system capacity.

Settling

Settling your nervous system, which is sometimes called *regulating* or *downshifting*, means you're shifting out of fight-or-flight mode and back down to a grounded state. Imagine confetti flying in the air and then gently settling down to the ground. In much the same way, you can settle your nervous system. As you settle, your cortisol levels drop, your heart rate decelerates, and you may notice other physical shifts in your body, too, such as muscles unclenching and peripheral vision returning, which are signs you feel safe again.

Doing any of the practices we just discussed (breathing, walking, time in nature, listening to music that supports regulation, etc.) can send signals of safety to your nervous system and help you settle faster.

Increasing Capacity

Your nervous system capacity is the amount of stress you can tolerate while still feeling safe and settled. Imagine a preschool teacher surrounded by screaming toddlers, bright colors, loud noises, mess, and clutter everywhere. Some people might find this environment extremely dysregulating! Yet, this teacher remains steady as a mountain even amid all the chaos. This is because she has developed an expansive nervous system capacity. In other words, it takes a *lot* to knock her into fight-or-flight mode.

You can increase your capacity, too—like blowing air into a balloon to make it bigger. How? By doing your favorite nervous system hygiene practice daily and consistently.

Dr. Elliott recommends choosing a nervous system hygiene practice that you enjoy and doing it 5–10 minutes a day for 21 days in a row. It can be breathwork, mindfulness, exercise, or other practices you find supportive. After 21 days, she says, you may notice some encouraging changes. Your capacity for handling stress increases, meaning it takes more to knock you off center. And when you do feel unsettled, your "bounceback-ability" (as Elliott calls it) is faster. You're able to return to a settled state quicker, rather than feeling derailed by a stressful event for hours.

When it comes to managing stress and anxiety, nervous system hygiene is the first and most important practice to build into your routine.

Prioritize Deep, Restorative Sleep

Poor sleep quality and sleep disturbances significantly increase the risk of developing anxiety and stress, and vice versa. However, the effect of poor sleep on anxiety is often stronger than the reverse, creating a vicious cycle where each worsens the other.[24,25]

Individuals with poor sleep quality are up to three to four times more likely to experience anxiety symptoms, and this association is observed across diverse populations, including women, students, and those with chronic stress.

On top of that, insufficient sleep has been linked to impaired reproductive hormone signaling and reduced ovarian reserve markers, which can negatively impact fertility.

Chapter 8 is dedicated to all things sleep-related, so we'll cover this topic thoroughly. But for starters, one powerful change you can make is to sync your body with the sun. Syncing up with the natural rhythm of the sun provides light and dark cues that retrain your brain and pineal gland to regulate hormones.[26] To sync up, here are the best practices to follow:

- **Great sleep starts in the morning:** Within 15–30 minutes of waking, get your eyes in natural light before screens. Ideally, step outside. If that's not doable, flood the room with sunlight.
- **Daylight exposure:** Spend time outdoors in the early morning and again in the evening without sunglasses, allowing natural light to reach your eyes (without ever looking directly at the sun). Midday is when your eyes most need protection, but early and late-day light are essential cues for your brain—helping it sense the angle and quality of sunlight that regulate your circadian rhythm.
- **Screen protection:** Wear blue-light-blocking glasses during screen time and try to avoid screens altogether in the hours leading up to bed.
- **Evening reset:** Take a walk at dusk/after dinner to signal the wind-down to your brain.

- **Dark nights:** Make your bedroom pitch black. If you can see your hand at arm's length, it's too bright.
- **Cool room:** When our bodies are hot, we will more easily wake out of a deep sleep. Keep your sleeping area at a comfortable, but coolish temperature.
- **Consistency:** Develop a consistent wake-up and wind-down routine that remains steady throughout the week. A steady routine allows your body to sync up with the sun more easily.

In addition to syncing with the sun, you can promote deeper sleep by engaging the senses with aromatherapy (especially lavender), calming music, and relaxation techniques (like a bedtime yoga or meditation practice). Consider sleep helpers, such as botanicals, amino acids, and specific nutrients, to help improve the quality of sleep. (More on this coming in Chapter 8.)

The more you protect your sleep like a prescription (consistent bedtime/wake time, morning light exposure, a cool/dark bedroom, and no late-night scrolling), the faster you'll see shifts in your energy, mood, immune health, metabolism, menstrual health, and overall nervous system resiliency.

Make Anti-Anxiety, Stress-Relieving Food Choices

The types of foods you eat and how you eat can either ramp up your physiologic stress or help support its regulation.

Blood sugar spikes and crashes amplify cortisol and adrenaline output. That's why a diet rich in fiber, protein, healthy fats, and micronutrients supports a steady stress response and reduces HPA axis overdrive.

Just like sleep, what and how you eat is such an important topic that it deserves its own chapter in *Hormone Powered*. More on this ahead. But for now, here's a quick guide on how to eat with stress management in mind. Here's a list of evidence-based eating choices you can make to help restore hormonal feedback between the brain, thyroid, adrenals, and ovaries, and manage your stress levels more effectively, rather than making things worse:

Anchor Meals with Protein[27]
Aim for 20–30 grams per meal. Protein stabilizes glucose and reduces adrenaline-driven crashes.

Pair Carbohydrates Wisely[28]
Combine carbohydrates with fiber and fat to slow absorption and prevent spikes.

Support the Gut-Brain Axis[29,30]
Incorporate fermented foods and prebiotic fibers. A balanced microbiome supports mood stability.

Eat Breakfast[31]
Skipping early nourishment can heighten cortisol output and anxiety sensitivity.

Reduce Stimulant Load[32,33]
Limit excess caffeine, refined sugar, and ultra-processed foods that destabilize blood sugar and inflammatory pathways.

Take Supplements with Stress-Managing Nutrients[34,35]
Higher intake of omega-3 fatty acids, magnesium, zinc, and selenium, as well as broad-spectrum micronutrients have been shown to lower anxiety.

Eat Enough
Align your caloric input to match your energetic output. Taking in adequate nourishment signals safety and sufficiency to your body.

Scan to download my three-week Anti-Anxiety Meal Plan—a free resource that my team and I created for you.

Use Botanical Medicine Helpers

Adding botanical medicine to your routine isn't a magical cure for stress and anxiety. But when you're already managing stress in other ways—doing your daily nervous system hygiene practices, getting deep sleep, and eating well—adding botanicals can give you an extra edge. That's why I call them "helpers." They're not a complete solution. But they can help to amplify the great work you're already doing.

For stress and anxiety, the two most helpful botanical groups are **nervines** and **adaptogens**.

Nervines

This class of herbs and plants includes several evidence-backed standouts known to calm the nervous system and restore resilience.

Chamomile (Matricaria recutita)[36]
A clinical study shows that taking capsules containing German chamomile extract (220–1,100 mg daily for eight weeks) reduces anxiety when compared with placebo in adult patients. Traditionally, chamomile has also been used to ease tension, support digestion, and promote gentle sleep.

Milky Oats (Avena sativa)[37]
Often used as a gentle nervine and nutritive tonic for the nervous system. Early clinical research shows promising effects on cognitive function and stress resilience, with some evidence for modulation of brain activity. Traditionally, it has been used to ease nervous exhaustion, decrease restlessness, and promote restorative sleep.

Skullcap (Scutellaria lateriflora)[38]
North American skullcap has a long history of use as a calming herb for anxiety, agitation, and insomnia. Preliminary clinical studies indicate it may enhance feelings of well-being and reduce anxiety without causing sedation or dependence. It appears to act on the GABA system in the brain, similar to how some pharmaceutical anxiolytics work, but in a gentler way.

Passionflower (Passiflora incarnata)[39]

Clinical research shows that taking a standardized extract reduces anxiety-associated symptoms. It is thought to work in part by increasing GABA activity in the brain, promoting a state of calm focus.

Lemon Balm (Melissa officinalis)[40]

Research shows that lemon balm use is comparable to some anxiolytics, and it is also used to improve effectiveness of certain conventional anti-anxiety medications. Traditionally, it has been used for nervousness, digestive upset, and sleep.

Want to boost your body's ability to handle stress? Look for a caffeine-free tea that includes one (or more) nervines like chamomile, milky oats, skullcap, passionflower, and lemon balm. Not a fan of tea? Try a tincture. My favorite brand for tea and tinctures are Herb Pharm, Gaia Herbs, and Mountain Rose Herbs.

Adaptogens

Adaptogens are botanicals that enhance the body's ability to adapt to stress, normalize physiological processes, and protect against stress-induced disorders.

Adaptogens modulate the HPA axis, reduce inflammation, and regulate neurotransmitters and stress hormones. Generally safe, but high doses or interactions with medications require caution and professional guidance.

Some adaptogens to consider:

Ashwagandha *(Withania somnifera)*[41,42]

Ashwagandha is a well-known adaptogen that helps reduce cortisol levels, improve sleep, and ease symptoms of anxiety and depression. Clinical studies show it can significantly reduce stress-related symptoms and enhance overall well-being through modulation of the HPA axis and GABAergic activity.

Rhodiola rosea[43,44]

Rhodiola supports the nervous system by improving stress adaptation, reducing fatigue, and enhancing mood. Clinical and preclinical research shows that it reduces symptoms of anxiety and depression and modulates neurotransmitter systems involved in emotional regulation.

Panax ginseng[45,46]

Panax ginseng enhances stress resilience, mental performance, and mood. Studies show it can reduce fatigue and improve quality of life in stressed individuals, with neuroprotective effects attributed to its ginsenosides, which modulate inflammatory and neuroendocrine pathways.

Siberian Ginseng *(Eleutherococcus senticosus)*[47]

Eleutherococcus is used to enhance stamina and stress resilience. It has shown benefits for mood and fatigue in older adults and demonstrates neuroprotective effects, including reducing damage from oxidative stress and supporting brain function.

Schisandra chinensis[48]

Schisandra helps regulate stress, improve mood, and support sleep. Research shows it reduces anxiety-like behaviors and supports the gut-brain axis, with active lignans such as schisandrin A–C contributing to its neuroprotective and adaptogenic effects.

Do Lab Testing

If anxiety feels disproportionate, persistent, or resistant to lifestyle shifts, look deeper.

Stress is emotional—but it is also biochemical.

In my clinic, we evaluate several key categories:

1. **Adrenal Function**

   Morning cortisol and diurnal rhythm patterns. Are you elevated all day? Flatlined? Reversed at night?

2. **Thyroid Panel**
   TSH, Free T4, Free T3, and thyroid antibodies. Even subtle dysfunction can present as anxiety, palpitations, and insomnia.
3. **Sex Hormones**
   Estradiol, progesterone, FSH/LH (cycle-timed when possible), and AMH when appropriate. Low luteal progesterone or fluctuating estrogen can heighten anxiety sensitivity—especially in perimenopause.
4. **Metabolic Markers**
   Fasting glucose, insulin, and A1c. Blood sugar instability can mimic or amplify anxiety through adrenaline surges.
5. **Nutrient Status**
   Vitamin D, ferritin, B12, folate, RBC magnesium. Deficiencies directly affect neurotransmitter production and nervous system stability.
6. **Inflammation + Gut Health**
   hs-CRP, homocysteine, and when indicated, comprehensive stool testing. The gut-brain axis is real and often overlooked.

When reviewing labs, look beyond "normal." Optimal ranges matter. Trends matter. Patterns matter.

Addressing underlying thyroid imbalance, adrenal dysregulation, nutrient depletion, or blood sugar instability can dramatically improve anxiety resilience.

Tracking Your Labs and Next Steps

If you haven't already done so, scan to download my Lab Testing Guide (another free resource for you), which has all the specifics regarding lab values, optimal ranges, and patterns that we look for in our clinic.

Bring your lab results to your naturopathic doctor, medical doctor, or other clinician with expertise in women's hormones to review your findings and create a personalized plan. Addressing physiologic contributors such as thyroid imbalance, adrenal stress, or nutrient deficiencies can significantly improve anxiety resilience and restore balance to your nervous system. Based on these results, talk to your ND, MD, or another endocrine-trained healthcare provider about next steps.

Specific Recommendations for the Caretaker, Achiever, and Survivor

So far, we have covered the universal stress management practices that I recommend for every woman, regardless of her Hormone Type.

No matter who you are, you need to find nervous system hygiene practices that you enjoy doing. You need to increase the amount of eustress (the good kind of stress) in your life while decreasing distress (the harmful variety). You need deep, restorative sleep and a diet that helps keep stress levels in check. (Check in with your dietary practices so that you are eating in a way that supports the stress response. Consider adding botanical medicine helpers into your routine.) Finally, I recommend lab testing for all women, too.

However, the Caretaker, Achiever, and Survivor each have their own hormonal patterns and different systems in the body that may be more heavily strained than others. So, I recommend a slightly different **stress management prescription** to each of my patients, depending on her type.

The Caretaker

Your Pattern: Highly sensitive nervous system. Prone to rumination. Easily knocked off center.

Your Three Highest-Leverage Moves

1. **Daily nervous system hygiene—non-negotiable.**
   Five to ten minutes of breathwork, a walk outside, or quiet connection before you give your energy to anyone else.
2. **Stabilize blood sugar + reduce stimulants.**
   Anchor meals with protein. Limit caffeine to one cup before noon. Replace afternoon caffeine with a calming herbal tea.
3. **Affirmation:**
   "When I regulate my nervous system, I change the emotional climate around me. My calm is powerful."

Why this works: The Caretaker's hormones stabilize when her nervous system feels safe. Regulation first. Everything else follows.

The Achiever

Your Pattern: High-output. Performance-driven. Prone to over-efforting and HPA axis strain.

Your Three Highest-Leverage Moves

1. **Reduce intensity; increase recovery.**
   Swap one high-intensity workout per week for restorative movement. Protect a defined stop time for work.
2. **Fuel adequately.**
   Avoid caloric deficit. Eat before and after workouts. Undereating amplifies cortisol.
3. **Affirmation:**
   "Progress comes from recovery, not more intensity. I can succeed without running on stress."

Why this works: The Achiever's hypothalamus is the conductor. When she signals safety through nourishment and recovery, cortisol quiets and hormones rebalance.

The Survivor

Your Pattern: Stress stored in the gut. History of inflammation, dysbiosis, or prolonged distress.

Your Three Highest-Leverage Moves

1. **Support digestion daily.**
   Add a 10-minute post-meal walk. Incorporate small amounts of probiotic and prebiotic foods gradually.
2. **Move stagnant stress out of the body.**
   Sweat two to three times per week through brisk walking, dancing, or sauna.
3. **Affirmation:**
   "My body has carried me through so much. I can rebuild resilience—gently and steadily."

Why this works: The Survivor's gut-brain axis drives her stress response. When digestion improves, mood and hormonal stability follow.

Bad Stress—Or the Good Kind? Sometimes, You Decide

Is it possible to switch distress (the bad kind of stress) into eustress (the beneficial kind) simply by changing the way you look at things? In other words, can you "decide" that a stressful situation is good for you, rather than harmful?

Not completely. But to some extent, yes, you do have this power within you. Research backs this up. I have seen this firsthand with the women I treat, and know, too.

When my colleague Alex was postpartum with a six-month-old baby, she got some terrible news: her 72-year-old mom had advanced stomach cancer, and the prognosis did not look good. Alex was shocked. Her mom was her best friend in the whole world, so this was devastating to say the least.

The next year was a complete blur, as Alex found herself thrust into a caregiver role for both her infant *and* mother.

Driving her mom to countless appointments. Talking to doctors and processing dizzying amounts of information. Helping her mom make life-or-death decisions. Holding her when she cried in pain. Alex took this on—while continuing to work full-time in her career, raise her baby, do nursing and pumping, and meet all the demands that go into caring for a very young child.

Was she tired? Absolutely. Were some days grueling and miserable? Yes. However, during this time, Alex made a conscious choice to view this experience as a temporary ordeal that would ultimately make her stronger. While experiencing what some might label distress, she chose to view it as eustress.

This story has a happy ending: her mom made a full recovery, is cancer free, and now swims in the ocean a mile or two every day. And, to some extent, Alex's decision to think about stress in a different way acted like a protective shield for her own body.

The Upside of Stress

Stanford psychologist Kelly McGonigal, author of *The Upside of Stress*, puts it like this: "When you change your mind about stress, you can change your body's response to stress.[49]"

In her TED Talk, "How to Make Stress Your Friend," McGonigal describes a Harvard study that found that viewing stress as "helpful" rather than "harmful" leads to a different physical response. When study participants were encouraged to interpret signs of stress as a "good" thing, their blood vessels relaxed and dilated, whereas those who thought about stress as "bad" were more likely to have constricted vessels.

I have observed this phenomenon with my own patients. Women who perceive perimenopause or menopause as "an exciting change" or "a beautiful new season of my life" or who think, "This change can be an opportunity to improve my health," tend to experience fewer unpleasant symptoms and have an easier transition overall. Studies back this up. As mentioned in one review of 13 studies on midlife women, "Women with more negative attitudes toward the menopause in general report more symptoms during the menopausal transition.[50]"

This doesn't mean you can snap your fingers and decide, "I'm experiencing the 'good' kind of stress!" It's not that simple. And sometimes, this just isn't true.

In an interview with *The Stanford Report*,[51] McGonigal explains that the goal isn't to pretend that chronic stress is good for you (it isn't) or lie about your feelings and pretend to feel cheerful when you don't. The real goal is to develop what she calls "protective beliefs" about stress.

Three Protective Beliefs

In the aforementioned Stanford interview, McGonigal elaborates on this, adding that "The three most protective beliefs about stress are: (1) to view your body's stress response as helpful, not debilitating—for example, to view stress as energy you can use; (2) to view yourself as able to handle, and even learn and grow from, the stress in your life; and (3) to view stress as something that everyone deals with, and not something that proves how uniquely screwed up you or your life is."

The point? Breathwork, gentle movement, botanicals including certain nervines and adaptogens—all of these can help protect your body against the negative impacts of stress. But your thoughts and beliefs can be protective, too.

Changing how you think about stress is easier when the other components of your wellness plan are already in place—particularly your support network. Going back to Alex, she was able to reframe a stressful experience in a more positive light thanks to her supportive husband and other family members, close friends, and therapist. If she had been alone? This experience might have broken her. But with support? It led to greater resilience. (This exemplifies why I place "Create Your Support Network" right at the center of your Hormone Action Plan. It is the core of it all, not an afterthought. Connection is power.)

Reframe

Is there a distressing situation in your life that you could reframe in a more positive light? How could this situation be helping you rather than hurting?

The point of this exercise is not to sugarcoat things but to challenge yourself to look at things from a new perspective. Reframing can shift your physiology and help protect your body from some of the harmful effects of stress.

Small Deposits, Exponential Returns

Managing stress and anxiety doesn't mean moving to a mountaintop monastery or off the grid—tempting as that might sound some days. It means weaving small but powerful practices into your daily life that tell your body, "You're safe now."

Breathing deeply for a few minutes. Going outside for a walk. Listening to calming, nervous system-regulating music. Coloring, knitting, or talking to a good friend. Sipping tea infused with botanical medicine helpers like chamomile or lemon balm. Looking at stressful events from a new perspective. Telling yourself a different story about what stress means, and your capacity to handle it.

These tiny, consistent actions compound over time. Like a long-term savings account, every small deposit into your nervous system today yields exponential returns when it comes to your hormones, mood, energy, and vitality now—and tomorrow.

What is one way you could tend to your nervous system and feel safe and settled, today?

Key Takeaways

- The first component of your Hormone Action Plan is managing stress and anxiety.
- Distress is the harmful kind of stress, which can throw your endocrine system out of whack and make it difficult for your hormones to do their jobs.
- Eustress is a beneficial kind of stress. When in small and intentional doses, eustress can make you stronger and more resilient.
- Your nervous systems' job is to scan your surroundings for potential threats, both physical and emotional.
- When a threat is detected, this system signals your body to shift into fight-or-flight mode. Hormones like epinephrine (otherwise known as adrenaline), norepinephrine, and cortisol get released, preparing your body for immediate action.
- Being in fight-or-flight mode for a short burst of time is fine. But being in this mode too often, or too long, has negative effects on your body.
- To manage stress and anxiety, the top five tools and practices are to:
  - Do daily nervous system hygiene
  - Prioritize deep, restorative sleep
  - Eat in a way that supports stress management
  - Use botanical medicine helpers
  - Do lab testing to check on the specific physiology that may be underneath your stress and anxiety
- Small deposits lead to exponential returns. By doing tiny practices consistently, you will notice a big shift in how you feel.
- The goal is not to eliminate stress from your life, but to increase your ability to handle it—which means adding more resources, tools, and support.

Notes

1. Kundaković, M., & Rocks, D. (2022). Sex Hormone Fluctuation and Increased Female Risk for Depression and Anxiety Disorders: From Clinical Evidence to Molecular Mechanisms. *Frontiers in Neuroendocrinology*. https://doi.org/10.1016/j.yfrne.2022.101010.
2. Leff-Gelman, P., et al. (2020). Cortisol and DHEA-S Levels in Pregnant Women with Severe Anxiety. *BMC Psychiatry*. https://doi.org/10.1186/s12888-020-02788-6.
3. Liang, G., et al. (2024). Menopause-Associated Depression: Impact of Oxidative Stress and Neuroinflammation on the Central Nervous System—A Review. *Biomedicines*. https://www.mdpi.com/2227-9059/12/1/184.
4. Farhane-Medina, N. Z., et al. (2022). Factors Associated with Gender and Sex Differences in Anxiety Prevalence and Comorbidity: A Systematic Review. *Science Progress*. https://journals.sagepub.com/doi/10.1177/00368504221135469.
5. Kowalczyk, M., et al. (2024). Differences in Anxiety, Worry, and Perceived Stress Among Naturally Cycling Women and Oral Contraceptives Users: A Cross-Sectional Study Investigating the Role of Contraceptive Types. https://link.springer.com/article/10.1007/s00737-023-01405-1.
6. Brouillard, A., et al. (2022). A Year Through the COVID-19 Pandemic: Deleterious Impact of Hormonal Contraception on Psychological Distress in Women. *Frontiers in Psychiatry*. https://www.frontiersin.org/journals/psychiatry/articles/10.3389/fpsyt.2022.835857/full.
7. Vigil, P., et al. (2022). Chronic Stress and Ovulatory Dysfunction: Implications in Times of COVID-19. https://www.frontiersin.org/journals/global-womens-health/articles/10.3389/fgwh.2022.866104/full.
8. Lu, S., et al. (2021). The Evolution of the Concept of Stress and the Framework of the Stress System. https://www.cell-stress.com/researcharticles/2021a-lu-cell-stress/.

9. Srinivasa, S. (2020). A Study on Different Types of Stress Among Women and Its Management. *International Journal of Trend in Scientific Research and Development*. https://www.ijtsrd.com/papers/ijtsrd31184.pdf.
10. Hall, M. H., et al. (2015). Chronic Stress Is Prospectively Associated with Sleep in Midlife Women: The SWAN Sleep Study. https://pubmed.ncbi.nlm.nih.gov/26039965/.
11. Matud, M. P. (2004). Gender Differences in Stress and Coping Styles. https://www.sciencedirect.com/science/article/abs/pii/S0191886904000200?via%3Dihub.
12. Palomba, S., et al. (2018). Lifestyle and Fertility: The Influence of Stress and Quality of Life on Female Fertility. https://rbej.biomedcentral.com/articles/10.1186/s12958-018-0434-y.
13. Skurat, K. (2023). 5 Ways to Turn Stress into Positive Stress and Productivity Fuel. *Calmerry*. https://calmerry.com/blog/stress/5-ways-to-turn-stress-into-a-productivity-fuel-and-use-it/.
14. Balban, M., et al. (2023). Brief Structured Respiration Practices Enhance Mood and Reduce Physiological Arousal. *Cell Reports Medicine*, 4. https://doi.org/10.1016/j.xcrm.2022.100895.
15. Lu, G., et al. (2021). Effects of Music Therapy on Anxiety: A Meta-Analysis of Randomized Controlled Trialso. https://www.sciencedirect.com/science/article/abs/pii/S0165178121004339?via%3Dihub.
16. Herold, F., et al. (2019). Functional and/or Structural Brain Changes in Response to Resistance Exercises and Resistance Training Lead to Cognitive Improvements—A Systematic Review. *European Review of Aging and Physical Activity*, 16. https://doi.org/10.1186/s11556-019-0217-2.
17. Yao, W., et al. (2020). The Effect of Exposure to the Natural Environment on Stress Reduction: A Meta-Analysis. *Urban Forestry & Urban Greening*, 126932. https://doi.org/10.1016/j.ufug.2020.126932.

18. Zawadzki, M., et al. (2015). Real-Time Associations Between Engaging in Leisure and Daily Health and Well-Being. *Annals of Behavioral Medicine*, 49, 605–615. https://doi.org/10.1007/s12160-015-9694-3.
19. Chin, M., & Kales, S. (2019). Understanding Mind-Body Disciplines: A Pilot Study of Breathing and Dynamic Muscle Contraction on Autonomic Nervous System Reactivity. *Stress and Health: Journal of the International Society for the Investigation of Stress*. https://doi.org/10.1002/smi.2887.
20. Choi, Y., et al. (2023). Emotional Freedom Technique Versus Written Exposure Therapy Versus Waiting List for Post-Traumatic Stress Disorder: Protocol for a Randomised Clinical MRI Study. https://bmjopen.bmj.com/content/13/6/e070389.
21. Subramaniam, S., et al. (2019). Massage Therapy for Anxiety Reduction: A Systematic Review. *Journal of Sports and Games*. https://doi.org/10.22259/2642-8466.0102003.
22. Kumari, D., & Patil, J. (2023). Guided Imagery for Anxiety Disorder: Therapeutic Efficacy and Changes in Quality of Life. *Industrial Psychiatry Journal*, 32, S191–S195. https://doi.org/10.4103/ipj.ipj_238_23.
23. Querstret, D., et al. (2020). Mindfulness-Based Stress Reduction and Mindfulness-Based Cognitive Therapy for Psychological Health and Well-Being in Nonclinical Samples: A Systematic Review and Meta-Analysis. *International Journal of Stress Management*. https://doi.org/10.1037/str0000165.
24. Peng, A., et al. (2024). The Bidirectional Relationship Between Sleep Disturbance and Anxiety: Sleep Disturbance Is a Stronger Predictor of Anxiety. https://www.sciencedirect.com/science/article/abs/pii/S1389945724003058?via%3Dihub.
25. Alwhaibi, M., & Al Aloola, N. A. (2023). Associations between Stress, Anxiety, Depression and Sleep Quality among Healthcare Students. https://www.mdpi.com/2077-0383/12/13/4340.

26. Robertson-Dixon, I., et al. (2023). The Influence of Light Wavelength on Human HPA Axis Rhythms: A Systematic Review. *Life*, 13. https://doi.org/10.3390/life13101968.
27. Norwitz, N. G., & Naidoo, U. (2021). Nutrition as Metabolic Treatment for Anxiety. *Frontiers in Psychiatry*. https://www.frontiersin.org/journals/psychiatry/articles/10.3389/fpsyt.2021.598119/full.
28. Aucoin, M., et al. (2021). Diet and Anxiety: A Scoping Review. https://www.mdpi.com/2072-6643/13/12/4418.
29. Ma, T., et al. (2021). Probiotic Consumption Relieved Human Stress and Anxiety Symptoms Possibly Via Modulating the Neuroactive Potential of the Gut Microbiota. https://www.sciencedirect.com/science/article/pii/S2352289521000023?via%3Dihub.
30. Liu, X., et al. (2024). Research Advance About Plant Polysaccharide Prebiotics, Benefit for Probiotics on Gut Homeostasis Modulation. https://www.sciencedirect.com/science/article/abs/pii/S221242922400261X?via%3Dihub.
31. Milajerdi, A. R., et al. (2017). The Relation Between Breakfast Consumption and Psychological Symptoms Among Adults. *Journal of Inflammatory Diseases*. https://www.researchgate.net/profile/Alireza-Milajerdi/publication/322007602_The_relation_between_breakfast_consumption_and_psychological_symptoms_among_adults/links/5a3d21c7458515f6b0399f53/The-relation-between-breakfast-consumption-and-psychological-symptoms-among-adults.pdf.
32. Sharma, S. (2024). Lifestyle and the Gut-Brain Axis Insights into Mental Health and Microbiome Interactions. https://www.ijisrt.com/lifestyle-and-the-gutbrain-axis-insights-into-mental-health-and-microbiome-interactions.
33. Sharma, S. (2024). Lifestyle and the Gut-Brain Axis Insights into Mental Health and Microbiome Interactions. *International Journal of Innovative Science and Research Technology*. https://www.ijisrt.com/lifestyle-and-the-gutbrain-axis-insights-into-mental-health-and-microbiome-interactions.

34. Wu, S.-X., et al. (2022). Possible Effects and Mechanisms of Dietary Natural Products and Nutrients on Depression and Anxiety: A Narrative Review. https://www.mdpi.com/2076-3921/11/11/2132.
35. Aucoin, M., et al. (2021). Diet and Anxiety: A Scoping Review. https://www.mdpi.com/2072-6643/13/12/4418.
36. Amsterdam, J. D., et al. (2009). A Randomized, Double-Blind, Placebo-Controlled Trial of Oral Matricaria Recutita (Chamomile) Extract Therapy for Generalized Anxiety Disorder. https://pubmed.ncbi.nlm.nih.gov/19593179/.
37. Kennedy, D. O., et al. (2020). Acute and Chronic Effects of Green Oat (Avena sativa) Extract on Cognitive Function and Mood During a Laboratory Stressor in Healthy Adults. https://pubmed.ncbi.nlm.nih.gov/32485993/.
38. Savage, K., et al. (2018). GABA-Modulating Phytomedicines for Anxiety: A Systematic Review of Preclinical and Clinical Evidence. https://pubmed.ncbi.nlm.nih.gov/29168225/.
39. Janda, K., et al. (2020). Passiflora Incarnata in Neuropsychiatric Disorders. https://pubmed.ncbi.nlm.nih.gov/33352740/.
40. Scholey, A., et al. (2014). Anti-Stress Effects of Lemon Balm-Containing Foods. *Nutrients*. https://pubmed.ncbi.nlm.nih.gov/25360512/.
41. Salve, J., et al. (2019). Adaptogenic and Anxiolytic Effects of Ashwagandha Root Extract in Healthy Adults: A Double-Blind, Randomized, Placebo-Controlled Clinical Study. https://pubmed.ncbi.nlm.nih.gov/32021735/.
42. Chandrasekhar, K., et al. (2012). A Prospective, Randomized Double-Blind, Placebo-Controlled Study of Safety and Efficacy of a High-Concentration Full-Spectrum Extract of Ashwagandha Root in Reducing Stress and Anxiety in Adults. *Indian Journal of Psychological Medicine*. https://pubmed.ncbi.nlm.nih.gov/23439798/.
43. Olsson, E. M., et al. (2009). A Randomised, Double-Blind, Placebo-Controlled, Parallel-Group Study of the Standardised Extract SHR-5 of the Roots of *Rhodiola rosea* in the Treatment of Subjects with Stress-Related Fatigue. *Planta Medica*.

44. Ishaque, S., et al. (2012). Rhodiola Rosea for Physical and Mental Fatigue: A Systematic Review. *BMC Complementary and Alternative Medicine*. https://pubmed.ncbi.nlm.nih.gov/22643043/.
45. Reay, J. L., et al. (2006). Effects of Panax Ginseng, Consumed With and Without Glucose, on Blood Glucose Levels and Cognitive Performance During Sustained 'Mentally Demanding' Tasks. *Journal of Psychopharmacology*. https://pubmed.ncbi.nlm.nih.gov/16401645/.
46. Kennedy, D. O., et al. (2001). Dose Dependent Changes in Cognitive Performance and Mood Following Acute Administration of Ginseng to Healthy Young Volunteers. https://pubmed.ncbi.nlm.nih.gov/11842896/.
47. Cicero, A. F. G., et al. (2004). Effects of Siberian ginseng (*Eleutherococcus senticosus*) in Elderly Hypertensive Volunteers: Mental Health and Social Functioning. https://pubmed.ncbi.nlm.nih.gov/15207399/.
48. Song, Y., et al. (2021). Raw and Wine Processed Schisandra chinensis Treatment Improved Anxiety- and Depression-Like Behavior Through Modulating Gut Microbiota Derivatives. https://www.sciencedirect.com/science/article/abs/pii/S0378874120333110?via%3Dihub.
49. "Kelly McGonigal: Can We Reframe The Way We Think About Stress?" National Public Radio (NPR). NPR. 2019. https://www.npr.org/transcripts/747384008.
50. Ayers, B., et al. (2010). The Impact of Attitudes Towards the Menopause on Symptom Experience. https://www.maturitas.org/article/S0378-5122(09)00397-1/fulltext.
51. "Embracing stress Is More Important Than Reducing Stress, Stanford Psychologist Says." Stanford News. Parker, C. B. 2015. https://news.stanford.edu/stories/2015/05/embracing-stress-is-more-important-than-reducing-stress,-stanford-psychologist-says.

Chapter 7

Stabilize Your Blood Sugar

When Mia came to see me, she was the picture of what most people would call "healthy." She meal-prepped on Sundays, tracked her workouts, and listened to every wellness podcast she could find. She was doing all the "right" things: intermittent fasting (which to her meant waiting until noon to start eating), cutting carbs, and squeezing in one more workout (an intense run or spin session) whenever she could.

And yet, she felt awful.

By midmorning, her mind was foggy, she was tired and irritable, and her hands were shaky. By 3 p.m., she was craving sugar so badly that she'd tear open her kids' snack drawer just to keep herself going. At night, she was exhausted but wired, lying awake with racing thoughts. Her period had become unpredictable, her sleep erratic, she was gaining weight and having a hard time losing it despite the efforts she was making, and her anxiety was starting to run the show.

She told me, "I feel like I'm doing everything I'm supposed to, but my body is rebelling. My doctor tells me my labs are normal, but I don't feel like myself." When we looked deeper, her labs were indeed in the "normal range," but as I explained to her, "Normal and optimal are not the same thing."

And when I analyzed her lab results more closely, they told the truth her body had been whispering for months. Her blood sugar was on a roller coaster, spiking after downing coffee and skipping breakfast, crashing midafternoon, and then soaring again after late-evening snacks—which she reached for to comfort herself after a long, exhausting day. Her insulin levels were climbing, her cortisol was high at the wrong times of the day, and her progesterone was almost nonexistent. **Her body wasn't broken. It was just out of rhythm.**

She had been living on stress hormones and caffeine instead of steady fuel. The very habits she believed were helping her "reset" her metabolism were, in fact, keeping her blood sugar and hormones locked in a constant tug of war.

Mia's story isn't rare. It's the modern woman's story.

So many women who are driven, health-conscious, busy, and multitasking are unknowingly destabilizing their hormones in the name of "wellness." We fast too long, sleep too little, live on caffeine and adrenaline, and wonder why we're fatigued, anxious, bloated, not ovulating, and feeling older and aging faster than we should be.

Once I show my patients how to manage their blood sugar effectively, they're often surprised by how effective this approach is—and what a life-changing difference it makes. Because when your blood sugar stabilizes, your hormones finally *exhale*. Your brain fog clears. You feel calmer and more energized. Your weight optimizes, and your body begins to settle into its natural balance. For those with cycles, things return to a healthy rhythm. For those seeking to conceive, they have a better chance of regular ovulation and maintaining a pregnancy. For those in perimenopause, their mood and weight hold steady rather than feeling erratic and out of control, and they feel more powerful during their transitional years: grounded, secure, and steady amid the changes.

This chapter is all about **stability**.

We'll explore one of the most overlooked but powerful keys to hormonal balance: your blood sugar rhythm.

Think of this chapter as your metabolic reset. It's not about dieting; it's about teaching your body to trust you again. When your blood sugar finds its rhythm, your hormones will follow.

What "Balanced Blood Sugar" Really Means

Balanced blood sugar means your glucose levels stay steady enough to fuel your brain, muscles, and cells—without excessive spikes or crashes.

Glucose is your body's primary energy source. Every time you think clearly, heal from a cut, ovulate, or build muscle, you're using glucose. It's the fuel that keeps your physiology moving forward.

When you eat, carbohydrates are broken down into glucose and released into your bloodstream. From there, your body decides: use it now, or store it for later. The goal is not to avoid glucose. The goal is to regulate it.

Balanced blood sugar, or glucose homeostasis, means your levels remain in a narrow range. Not too high or too low. Just steady.

The Blood Sugar Duo: Insulin and Glucagon

Two hormones run this system: insulin and glucagon.

After you eat, insulin is released from the pancreas. Its job is to escort glucose into your cells and signal storage. Insulin is the only hormone that lowers blood sugar.

When you haven't eaten for several hours and blood sugar begins to fall, glucagon steps in. It signals the liver to release stored glucose back into circulation.

Think of insulin and glucagon as partners balancing a seesaw. One lowers. One raises. Together, they keep your energy stable.

Other hormones—like cortisol, adrenaline, thyroid hormones, growth hormone, and IGF-1—also influence blood sugar, especially during stress or fasting. Hormones never work alone. When blood sugar is unstable, the ripple effects travel quickly:

- Chronically high insulin can raise testosterone and suppress progesterone.
- Chronically low blood sugar can drive cortisol and shut down ovulation.

Blood sugar balance is not separate from hormone balance. It is hormone balance.

Blood Sugar Through the Years

Blood sugar regulation in women changes significantly during puberty, pregnancy, postpartum, perimenopause, and menopause, primarily due to hormonal shifts, especially in estrogen and insulin sensitivity.

The following sections cover how the blood sugar story unfolds through the different seasons of a woman's life, and some of the issues that can arise at certain times.

Puberty[1,2,3]

During puberty, insulin sensitivity temporarily decreases. Growth hormone, IGF-1, and rising sex steroids create a natural, short-lived state of insulin resistance. In healthy teens, the pancreas compensates and blood sugar remains stable.

When nutrition is poor or weight increases significantly, that temporary shift can become more problematic.

Pregnancy and Postpartum[4,5,6]

Pregnancy intentionally increases insulin resistance, especially in the third trimester. This ensures a steady glucose supply to the developing baby.

Most women compensate well. Some do not, resulting in gestational diabetes.

After delivery, insulin sensitivity typically improves quickly. However, women who experienced gestational diabetes remain at higher long-term risk for metabolic dysfunction.

Perimenopause and Menopause[7,8,9]

As estrogen declines, insulin sensitivity decreases. Many women notice rising fasting glucose, increased abdominal fat, and more volatile energy patterns.

Menopausal hormone therapy can sometimes support metabolic stability, but it must be individualized.

Major hormonal transitions are like walking across a suspension bridge instead of solid ground. Balance is still possible—but it requires more intention.

The following table shows insulin sensitivity throughout stages of life.

Life Stage	Insulin Sensitivity	Key Hormonal Changes	Glucose Regulation Impact
Puberty[a,b,c]	↓ (then recovers)	↑ Growth hormone (GH), IGF-1, sex steroids (estrogen, androgens)	Temporary insulin resistance (a normal physiological adaptation that recovers after puberty)
Pregnancy[d,e,f,g]	↓ (especially late pregnancy)	↑ Placental hormones (hPL, progesterone, cortisol, estrogen)	Increased insulin resistance to provide glucose to the fetus; risk of gestational diabetes if compensation inadequate

Life Stage	Insulin Sensitivity	Key Hormonal Changes	Glucose Regulation Impact
Postpartum[h,i,j,k]	↑ (improves after delivery)	↓ Placental hormones	Rapid improvement in insulin sensitivity; possible persistent dysregulation or future type 2 diabetes risk if gestational diabetes occurred
Menopause[l,m,n,o]	↓	↓ Estrogen	Increased insulin resistance, impaired insulin secretion, higher fasting and post-meal glucose, more glycemic variability, greater type 2 diabetes risk

[a] Bloch, C., et al. (1987). Puberty Decreases Insulin Sensitivity. *The Journal of Pediatrics*, 110 3, 481–487. https://doi.org/10.1016/s0022-3476(87)80522-x.

[b] Goran, M., & Gower, B. (2001). Longitudinal Study on Pubertal Insulin Resistance. *Diabetes*, 50 11, 2444–2550. https://doi.org/10.2337/diabetes.50.11.2444.

[c] Littlejohn, E., et al. (2006). 12 Both Insulin Sensitivity and Disposition Index Fall During Normal Female Puberty Without a Change in Glucose Tolerance. *Pediatric Research*, 60, 492–492. https://doi.org/10.1203/00006450-200610000-00034.

[d] Waters, T., et al. (2019). Longitudinal Changes in Glucose Metabolism in Women With Gestational Diabetes, From Late Pregnancy to the Postpartum Period. *Diabetologia*, 63, 385–394. https://doi.org/10.1007/s00125-019-05051-0.

[e] Dratver, M., et al. (2021). Longitudinal Changes in Glucose During Pregnancy in Women With Gestational Diabetes Risk Factors. *Diabetologia*, 65, 541–551. https://doi.org/10.1007/s00125-021-05622-0.

[f] Chen, Y., et al. (2024). Gestational and Postpartum Exposure to PM2.5 Components and Glucose Metabolism in Chinese Women: A Prospective Cohort Study. *Environmental Science & Technology*. https://doi.org/10.1021/acs.est.4c03087.

[g] Phaloprakarn, C., & Tangjitgamol, S. (2020). Glucose Levels During Gestational Diabetes Pregnancy and the Risk of Developing Postpartum Diabetes or Prediabetes. *BMC Pregnancy and Childbirth*, 22. https://doi.org/10.1186/s12884-021-04352-w.

[h] Waters, T., et al. (2019). Longitudinal Changes in Glucose Metabolism in Women With Gestational Diabetes, From Late Pregnancy to the Postpartum Period. *Diabetologia*, 63, 385–394. https://doi.org/10.1007/s00125-019-05051-0.

[i] Phaloprakarn, C., & Tangjitgamol, S. (2020). Glucose Levels During Gestational Diabetes Pregnancy and the Risk of Developing Postpartum Diabetes or Prediabetes. *BMC Pregnancy and Childbirth*, 22. https://doi.org/10.1186/s12884-021-04352-w.

[j] Ding, Y., et al. (2022). Intrapartum and early postpartum glycemic profiles in women with gestational diabetes mellitus: an observational study. *Chinese Medical Journal*, 135, 2547–2553. https://doi.org/10.1097/cm9.0000000000002423.
[k] Arnoriaga-Rodríguez, M., et al. (2023). Modifiable Risk Factors and Trends in Changes in Glucose Regulation during the First Three Years Postdelivery: The St Carlos Gestational Diabetes Mellitus Prevention Cohort. *Nutrients*, 15. https://doi.org/10.3390/nu15234995.
[l] Bermingham, K., et al. (2022). Menopause Is Associated With Postprandial Metabolism, Metabolic Health and Lifestyle: The ZOE PREDICT study. *eBioMedicine*, 85. https://doi.org/10.1016/j.ebiom.2022.104303.
[m] Zhu, J., et al. (2023). Role of estrogen in the regulation of central and peripheral energy homeostasis: from a menopausal perspective. *Therapeutic Advances in Endocrinology and Metabolism*, 14. https://doi.org/10.1177/20420188231199359.
[n] Tramunt, B., et al. (2019). Sex differences in metabolic regulation and diabetes susceptibility. *Diabetologia*, 63, 453–461. https://doi.org/10.1007/s00125-019-05040-3.
[o] Lambrinoudaki, I., et al. (2022). The Interplay Between Diabetes Mellitus and Menopause: Clinical Implications. *Nature Reviews Endocrinology*, 18, 608–622. https://doi.org/10.1038/s41574-022-00708-0.

The Hormonal Cost of Blood Sugar Imbalance

Blood sugar balance is hormone balance. Every meal, every night's sleep, every bout of stress is a signal your hormones listen to.

When blood sugar is chronically high, insulin rises. When insulin remains elevated for too long:

- Inflammation rises.
- Androgens increase.
- Progesterone can fall.
- Ovulation becomes inconsistent.

This pattern often shows up as premenstrual syndrome (PMS), acne, hair thinning, irregular cycles, or polyendocrine metabolic ovarian syndrome (PMOS) progression.

When blood sugar drops too low, cortisol surges to compensate. Over time, this stress response can disrupt thyroid conversion, suppress ovulation, and amplify anxiety.

Hormonal transitions as mentioned—puberty, pregnancy, postpartum, perimenopause—naturally increase metabolic vulnerability. If foundational rhythms are weak, these seasons magnify imbalance.

But with steady fuel, restorative sleep, muscle-building movement, and nervous system regulation, stability is possible and predictable.

Let's Talk About Insulin Resistance

I gave a quick definition of "insulin resistance" earlier in this chapter. But it's such an important concept—with such a massive impact on your well-being—that it deserves its own section.

Think of insulin as a key. Its job is to unlock your cells so glucose can enter and be used as fuel.

In a healthy system, the key turns easily. You eat, insulin rises briefly, glucose enters your cells, and blood sugar returns to baseline.

But when blood sugar is elevated too often, for too long, the locks begin to stick. Your cells become less responsive. The key still fits—but it doesn't work as smoothly.

Your pancreas compensates by producing more insulin to force the door open.

For a while, blood sugar stays "normal." But insulin levels quietly climb. This is how insulin resistance develops—years before prediabetes or type 2 diabetes show up on a standard lab test.

That's why fasting insulin is often more revealing than glucose alone.

The good news? Early insulin resistance is highly reversible. When we reduce inflammatory inputs—chronic stress, sleep disruption, excess refined carbohydrates—and build muscle, improve nutrient status, and stabilize meals, those locks regain sensitivity.

The key works again.

And when insulin works efficiently, your entire hormonal ecosystem stabilizes.

Five Science-Backed Lifestyle and Dietary Tools to Balance Blood Sugar

1. Anchor Your Meals with Protein (20–30g per Meal)

Protein slows the release of glucose into your bloodstream, keeping your energy and mood steady while improving satiety and reducing cravings. Studies consistently show that high-protein and Mediterranean-style diets improve insulin sensitivity and glycemic control and even reduce insulin resistance in women with PMOS, obesity, and metabolic syndrome.[10,11,12,13]

Aim for at least 20–30 grams of protein per meal (think: eggs, salmon, lentils, tempeh, hemp hearts, or Greek yogurt).

One simple but powerful trick: eat in the right order. Start with your vegetables, protein, and high-fiber foods first; then finish with starchy carbohydrates. This might look like starting with a veggie-packed salad, salmon, and a sprinkle of fiber-rich flax seeds on top, followed by a more carbohydrate-dense food like a baked sweet potato or scoop of rice. Research in women with gestational diabetes shows this "food sequencing" can blunt post-meal glucose and insulin spikes.[14] It's one of the simplest, most research-supported habits for blood sugar stability. And it's great news for women who love carbs—you don't need to cut them out. Just swap processed carbs for higher-quality options and change the sequencing of when you eat them.

2. Eat Fiber Like Your Hormones Depend on It (Because They Do)

Fiber does far more than support digestion; it's essential hormone therapy.

Soluble and insoluble fibers from foods like flax, chia, pumpkin seeds, sesame seeds, sunflower seeds, leafy greens, and legumes help regulate glucose absorption, feed your gut microbiome, and enhance estrogen metabolism via the estrobolome (the gut's estrogen-processing bacteria).

High-fiber, low-glycemic-index diet eating patterns are strongly associated with improved fasting and post-meal glucose levels and even reduced insulin requirements in women with gestational diabetes.[15]

Seeds like pumpkin, flax, and hemp also supply magnesium, one of the most common nutrient deficiencies in women. Magnesium plays a crucial role in glucose metabolism and insulin receptor sensitivity, and higher dietary intake is linked with a lower risk of developing diabetes.[16]

Try this: add a tablespoon of ground flax, chia, and/or pumpkin seeds to your morning smoothie, and include a hearty dose of greens or legumes (like beans, peas, lentils, and chickpeas) with lunch and dinner.

All About Seed Cycling

Want to supercharge your results? Try seed cycling. This means timing when you eat certain high-fiber, nutrient-dense seeds to correspond with the different phases of your menstrual cycle.[17]

How does seed cycling work? During the first half of your cycle (Day 1 through ovulation), consume 1 tablespoon each of ground flax and pumpkin seeds daily. During the second half (post-ovulation through Day 28), rotate to 1 tablespoon each of sesame and sunflower seeds. If your cycle is irregular, simply rotate every two weeks. If you are not cycling, you may still rotate in two-week intervals.

The rationale? Flax and pumpkin contain lignans and phytoestrogen compounds that may support healthy estrogen signaling and ovulatory patterns. Sesame and sunflower provide minerals and anti-inflammatory nutrients that may support the luteal phase.

Is there research to support seed cycling? The answer is yes and no. There is a small study evaluating seed cycling and menstrual-related symptoms including mood, period pain, breast tenderness, and digestion with most participants reporting improvement.[18]

At the same time, large-scale clinical trials on seed cycling as a structured protocol are absent. What we do have is meaningful research supporting the metabolic, anti-inflammatory, and hormone-modulating properties of the individual seeds themselves.

My recommendation: if seed cycling is something you're curious to try, go for it and see if it works for you.

3. Move Your Body—Especially After Meals

Just like protein and fiber, movement is another key to blood sugar balance. You don't need to overtrain; you just need to move! A 10-minute walk at a moderate, gentle pace immediately after a meal can lower post-meal blood glucose by anywhere from 12–30% and improve how efficiently your muscles use glucose for energy.[19,20]

Both aerobic exercise (like brisk walking or cycling) and resistance training (like lifting weights or bodyweight exercises) improve insulin sensitivity and reduce insulin requirements, even in women with gestational diabetes.[21,22,23,24]

Tip: Walk after meals when you can. If you can't go outside, try a walking pad, treadmill, march in place, or stroll around indoors for 10 minutes. (Yes, walking from the kitchen to the bedroom to your home office totally counts.) If you're short on time and don't have 10 minutes to spare, try exercise snacks—short, intentional bursts of activity like climbing one flight of stairs, doing 10 squats, or stretching for one minute after eating. When it comes to balancing your blood sugar, any movement, however brief, is better than none.

I want to give a special shout-out to resistance training, which is especially powerful for women in the perimenopause and menopause years. Why? Because starting around age 30, you start to lose 3–5% of your muscle mass[25] every decade until the end of your life. While this gradual attrition is a natural part of aging, inactivity and hormonal imbalances can accelerate the process, causing you to lose more muscle mass, faster than you ought to.

The remedy? Resistance training to increase muscle mass via a process called *muscle hypertrophy*, where existing muscle fibers grow larger and stronger. Resistance training, also known as *strength training*, can look like lifting weights at the gym, doing a workout with elastic resistance bands or TRX straps, or simply lifting heavy items throughout your day—kids, grandkids, grocery bags, shoveling piles of snow from your driveway, and other no-gym-required-workouts.

What's the connection between muscle and insulin? To quote Alisa Bowman in an article for the Mayo Clinic Press, "Muscle tissue secretes substances that encourage cells to use blood sugar more efficiently [...] As a result, bigger, stronger muscles can help reduce the risk of insulin resistance and type 2 diabetes.[26]" So, getting toned muscles isn't just about aesthetics or vanity—it's a powerful choice to keep your blood sugar, and hormones, in balance.

On a related note, if weight loss is part of your wellness plan, know that even a 5–10% reduction in body weight through a balanced diet and exercise can significantly improve insulin resistance, too.[27,28]

4. Prioritize Sleep During the Key Hormonal Repair Hours: 10 p.m. to 6 a.m.

Sleep is one of the most underrated tools for metabolic and hormonal health. Poor sleep raises cortisol and glucose overnight, decreases leptin (the satiety hormone), and increases ghrelin (the hunger hormone), setting off a vicious cycle of cravings and energy crashes.

Research consistently links insufficient or irregular sleep to higher insulin resistance, increased appetite, and difficulty maintaining a healthy weight. The hours between 10 p.m. and 6 a.m. are your body's natural repair window, when growth hormone peaks, cells restore insulin sensitivity, and the nervous system recalibrates.

Stick to consistent bed and wake times (even on weekends) and keep screens and bright lights off an hour before bed to protect melatonin, your sleep hormone. You'll wake up feeling more refreshed—and you're helping to stabilize your blood sugar levels and hormones for the day ahead. (More on this in the next chapter, which is all about deep, restorative sleep.)

5. Manage Stress Like It's Metabolic Medicine

Cortisol, the main stress hormone, directly raises blood sugar. When cortisol stays elevated for too long, it signals your liver to release more glucose, which, over time, can worsen insulin resistance.

Research increasingly recognizes chronic stress and poor autonomic regulation as major drivers of metabolic dysfunction. This is especially true for women juggling high workloads, caretaking roles, or disrupted sleep patterns.

To counteract the negative effects of stress, remember to do your daily nervous system hygiene (head back to Chapter 6 for a quick refresher course on managing stress and anxiety), which are simple practices that retrain your body to feel safe and supported: breathwork practices, morning sunlight exposure, grounding, walking in nature, journaling, or any activity that gets you out of your head and into your body.

Mind-body and relaxation techniques, including yoga and mindfulness, have been shown to lower fasting glucose and cortisol levels while improving insulin sensitivity in women.[29]

Treat stress regulation as seriously as your nutrition plan. It's the lever that keeps every other system, especially your blood sugar, steady.

Rhythm, Not Rigidity

Here's the main takeaway from the five tips I just shared: balancing blood sugar is about rhythm, not rigidity. The most effective strategies for women are the ones that build consistency: balanced, protein-rich meals, fiber-forward foods, regular movement, restorative sleep, and calm within your nervous system. Together, these habits form the foundation of metabolic resilience and hormonal peace.

Reflect

- When during the day do you feel most tired, feel wired, or crave sugar?
- How often do you skip meals or caffeinate on an empty stomach?
- What's one small change you can make, starting today, to keep your blood sugar levels steadier?

(Remember, it can be as small as "eating protein before carbs" or "moving gently for 10 minutes after a meal" or "getting to sleep before 10 p.m." Research confirms: tiny adjustments like these *do* make a difference.)

Supplements That Support Metabolic Health

When it comes to keeping your blood sugar in balance and preventing insulin resistance, I recommend starting with the five lifestyle changes that we just covered. However, if you're already practicing those habits and want to give your body an additional boost, see Table 7.1 for the most studied and effective nutrients for blood sugar balance, and see Table 7.2 for the botanical helpers.

Before adding these supplements to your diet, especially if you are pregnant, breastfeeding, or taking any medications, talk to your naturopathic physician or another healthcare provider.

Table 7.1 Top Nutrients and Supplements for Blood Sugar Support

Nutrient/ Botanical/ Supplement	Evidence for Blood Sugar Support	Key Mechanisms
Chromium[p]	Strongest evidence for lowering fasting glucose and insulin resistance	Enhances insulin action
Vitamin D[q]	Effective for reducing HbA1c, fasting glucose, and insulin resistance	Modulates insulin secretion and sensitivity, lowers inflammation
Vitamin C and vitamin E[r]	Reduces oxidative stress, may lower fasting glucose and HbA1c	Antioxidant and anti-inflammatory
Zinc and magnesium[s]	Reduces HbA1c and fasting glucose	Required for insulin synthesis, storage, and secretion
Selenium[t]	Some positive results with caution at higher doses	Antioxidant, may modulate insulin pathways
Omega-3 fatty acids[u]	Modest glycemic effect; stronger on inflammation and lipids	Anti-inflammatory, improves membrane function
Alpha-lipoic acid[v]	Improves insulin sensitivity and oxidative stress markers	Potent antioxidant, supports mitochondrial function
Myo-inositol and D-chiro-inositol[w,x]	Improves blood sugar stability, insulin resistance, improve in women, especially for GDM and PMOS, with strong safety and efficacy profiles	Acts as insulin sensitizers by enhancing insulin signaling and increases glucose transporter type 4 (GLUT4) translocation to the cell membrane
Coenzyme Q10[y]	May improve HbA1c and fasting glucose	Antioxidant, mitochondrial support
Probiotics, prebiotics[z]	May improve glycemic control and insulin sensitivity	Modulate gut microbiota and endotoxemia

[p] Xia, J., et al. (2023). Comparative Effects of Vitamin and Mineral Supplements in the Management of Type 2 Diabetes in Primary Care: A Systematic Review and Network Meta-Analysis of Randomized Controlled Trials. *Pharmacological Research*, 106647. https://doi.org/10.1016/j.phrs.2023.106647.

[q] Kazemi, A., et al. (2022). Comparison of Nutritional Supplements for Glycemic Control in Type 2 Diabetes: A Systematic Review and Network Meta-Analysis of Randomized Trials. *Diabetes Research and Clinical Practice*, 110037. https://doi.org/10.1016/j.diabres.2022.110037.

[r] Fong, C., et al. (2022). Efficacy and Safety of Nutrient Supplements for Glycaemic Control and Insulin Resistance in Type 2 Diabetes: An Umbrella Review and Hierarchical Evidence Synthesis. *Nutrients*, 14. https://doi.org/10.3390/nu14112295.

[s] Kazemi, A., et al. (2022). Comparison of Nutritional Supplements for Glycemic Control in Type 2 Diabetes: A Systematic Review and Network Meta-Analysis of Randomized Trials. *Diabetes Research and Clinical Practice*, 110037. https://doi.org/10.1016/j.diabres.2022.110037.

[t] Ouyang, J., et al. (2022). Potential Benefits of Selenium Supplementation in Reducing Insulin Resistance in Patients with Cardiometabolic Diseases: A Systematic Review and Meta-Analysis. *Nutrients*, 14. https://doi.org/10.3390/nu14224933.

[u] Kazemi, A., et al. (2022). Comparison of Nutritional Supplements for Glycemic Control in Type 2 Diabetes: A Systematic Review and Network Meta-Analysis of Randomized Trials. *Diabetes Research and Clinical Practice*, 110037. https://doi.org/10.1016/j.diabres.2022.110037.

[v] Lei, L., et al. (2016). Alpha-Lipoic Acid Attenuates Endoplasmic Reticulum Stress-Induced Insulin Resistance by Improving Mitochondrial Function in HepG2 Cells. *Cellular Signalling*, 28, 10, 1441–1450. https://doi.org/10.1016/j.cellsig.2016.06.024.

[w] Pustotina, O., et al. (2024). The Effects of Myo-Inositol and D-Chiro-Inositol in a Ratio 40:1 on Hormonal and Metabolic Profile in Women with Polyendocrine Metabolic Ovarian Syndrome Classified as Phenotype A by the Rotterdam Criteria and EMS-Type 1 by the EGOI Criteria. *Gynecologic and Obstetric Investigation*, 89, 131–139. https://doi.org/10.1159/000536163.

[x] Celentano, C., et al. (2020). The Influence of Different Inositol Stereoisomers Supplementation in Pregnancy on Maternal Gestational Diabetes Mellitus and Fetal Outcomes in High-Risk Patients: A Randomized Controlled Trial. *The Journal of Maternal-Fetal & Neonatal Medicine*, 33, 743–751. https://doi.org/10.1080/14767058.2018.1500545.

[y] Liang, Y., et al. (2022). Effects of Coenzyme Q10 Supplementation on Glycemic Control: A GRADE-Assessed Systematic Review and Dose-Response Meta-Analysis of Randomized Controlled Trials. *eClinicalMedicine*, 52. https://doi.org/10.1016/j.eclinm.2022.101602.

[z] Fong, C., et al. (2022). Efficacy and Safety of Nutrient Supplements for Glycaemic Control and Insulin Resistance in Type 2 Diabetes: An Umbrella Review and Hierarchical Evidence Synthesis. *Nutrients*, 14. https://doi.org/10.3390/nu14112295.

Table 7.2 Most Studied Botanicals for Blood Sugar Support

Botanical	Primary Findings for Glycemic Control	Key Notes
Cinnamon *(Cinnamomum cassia/verum)*[aa]	Lowers fasting glucose and improves insulin sensitivity in several trials	Dose and species vary across studies
Bitter melon *(Momordica charantia)*[bb]	Insulin-like activity, lowers glucose in some trials	Formulation and ripeness affect potency
Fenugreek *(Trigonella foenum-graecum)*[cc]	Improves postprandial control and insulin sensitivity	Often used as seed powder or standardized extract
Berberine[dd]	Comparable to some oral agents for lowering glucose and improving HOMA-IR	Check for drug interactions; GI side effects possible
Aloe vera, ginseng, Gymnema, nopal, garlic[ee]	Hypoglycemic effects reported in clinical or preclinical work	Evidence heterogeneous across preparations
Curcumin *(turmeric)*[ff]	Antioxidant and anti-inflammatory; may improve insulin sensitivity	Bioavailability depends on formulation
Quercetin, rutin, polyphenols[gg]	Flavonoids with antioxidant and glucose-lowering properties	Mechanisms include AMPK activation and reduced inflammation

[aa] Moridpour, A., et al. (2023). The Effect of Cinnamon Supplementation on Glycemic Control in Patients with Type 2 Diabetes Mellitus: An Updated Systematic Review and Dose-Response Meta-Analysis of Randomized Controlled Trials. *Phytotherapy Research*, 38, 117–130. https://doi.org/10.1002/ptr.8026.

[bb] Gao, Y., et al. (2021). Bitter Melon and Diabetes Mellitus. *Food Reviews International*, 39, 618–638. https://doi.org/10.1080/87559129.2021.1923733.

[cc] Shabil, M., et al. (2023). Effect of Fenugreek on Hyperglycemia: A Systematic Review and Meta-Analysis. *Medicina*, 59. https://doi.org/10.3390/medicina59020248.

[dd] Wang, J., et al. (2024). Effects of Administering Berberine Alone or in Combination on Type 2 Diabetes Mellitus: A Systematic Review and Meta-Analysis. *Frontiers in Pharmacology*, 15. https://doi.org/10.3389/fphar.2024.1455534.

[ee] Ota, A., & Ulrih, N. (2017). An Overview of Herbal Products and Secondary Metabolites Used for Management of Type Two Diabetes. *Frontiers in Pharmacology*, 8. https://doi.org/10.3389/fphar.2017.00436.

[ff] Ridho, M., & Indriani, R. (2025). The Potential of Curcuma longa as an Antidiabetic Agent: Review. *Journal of Medicine and Health Technology*. https://doi.org/10.12962/j30466865.v2i1.2383.

[gg] Zielinska, D., et al. (2025). Multifaceted Biological Activity of Rutin, Quercetin, and Quercetin's Glucosides. *Molecules*, 30. https://doi.org/10.3390/molecules30122555.

When Your Body Whispers, Get Tested

If you're struggling with fatigue, cravings, brain fog, irritability, or stubborn weight gain, I strongly encourage you to get your lab testing done. These are often early signals of blood sugar and insulin dysregulation.

Glucose imbalance develops quietly, sometimes years before prediabetes appears on routine screening. Strategic lab testing allows us to catch patterns early, when they are still highly reversible.

Here are the most useful markers.

Which Tests to Do

Core Metabolic Markers

Fasting Glucose + Fasting Insulin

This pairing is foundational.

Optimal fasting glucose: 75–85 mg/dL

Optimal fasting insulin: under 8 μIU/mL

Glucose can remain "normal" while insulin climbs. Elevated fasting insulin is often the earliest sign of insulin resistance.

HbA1c

Reflects your three-month blood sugar average.

For metabolic and hormone health, I prefer to see levels under 5.2%, even if the normal lab range extends higher.

Lipid Panel

Insulin resistance often shows up as:

- High triglycerides
- Low HDL
- Triglyceride-to-HDL ratio above 2:1

These shifts can appear before glucose changes.

Comprehensive Metabolic Panel (CMP)

Provides insight into liver enzymes and metabolic strain. Elevated AST or ALT can signal fatty liver or insulin-related stress.

Hormone Stress Markers

Cortisol (morning or diurnal pattern)

Chronically elevated cortisol raises blood sugar. A flattened or reversed curve may reflect nervous system dysregulation.

Thyroid Panel (TSH, Free T4, Free T3, Reverse T3)

Thyroid hormones regulate metabolic rate and glucose uptake. Even mild thyroid dysfunction can worsen insulin resistance.

Sex Hormones (Estradiol, Progesterone, Testosterone, SHBG)

Insulin resistance lowers SHBG and can increase free testosterone—particularly in PMOS and perimenopause.

- Estradiol + FSH/LH: ideally tested Days 2–5
- Progesterone: 5–7 days post-ovulation
- Testosterone + SHBG: any cycle day

Foundational Nutrients

Vitamin D (goal often above 50 ng/mL)

RBC Magnesium + RBC Zinc

Ferritin (ideally not too low or excessively high)

These nutrients directly influence insulin signaling and glucose metabolism.

Omega-3 Index

Above 5% is associated with improved insulin sensitivity and lower inflammation.

Gut Health

The microbiome influences glucose metabolism and inflammation. Dysbiosis can worsen insulin resistance. Comprehensive stool testing can uncover inflammatory or microbial drivers.

What We're Looking For

Early metabolic strain may look like:

- Fasting glucose above 90 mg/dL
- Fasting insulin above 5 μIU/mL
- HbA1c creeping above 5.2%
- Elevated triglycerides or TG:HDL ratio above 2
- Low SHBG or elevated free testosterone
- Low vitamin D or magnesium
- Flattened cortisol curve

These are early warning signals, not diagnoses.

Why This Matters

These labs are more than numbers; they're your body's communication system. When we identify insulin resistance, nutrient depletion, inflammation, or stress dysregulation early, we can reverse course with lifestyle, targeted supplementation, and, when appropriate, conventional tools.

Specific Recommendations for the Caretaker, Achiever, and Survivor

Every woman benefits from consistent meals anchored with protein, fiber, and healthy fats; daily post-meal movement; a stable sleep window between 10 p.m. and 6 a.m.; and simple nervous system hygiene. But, depending on whether you're a Caretaker, Achiever, or Survivor, you can tweak your approach to align with your Hormone Type. The following are my recommendations.

The Caretaker

Your Pattern: Caretakers destabilize blood sugar by under-fueling and over-giving. Their system runs on cortisol and caffeine instead of steady nourishment.

Your Three Highest-Leverage Moves

1. **Eat protein before caffeine.**
   Within 30–60 minutes of waking, anchor your body with 20–30 grams of protein before coffee or matcha. This single shift stabilizes cortisol, glucose, and afternoon energy.
2. **Stabilize meals before intensity.**
   Three consistent meals and one simple protein-forward snack daily. Build muscle gradually with low-to-moderate resistance training instead of pushing through exhaustion.
3. **Affirmation:**
   "I nourish myself first so I can show up fully for others."

Why this works: The Caretaker's blood sugar instability is driven by depletion. Stability begins with appropriate fuel and nourishment.

The Achiever

Your Pattern: Achievers destabilize blood sugar through intensity—overtraining, under-fueling, fasting too long, riding adrenaline.

Your Three Highest-Leverage Moves

1. **Cap your fast at 12–13 hours.**
   No extended fasting. Eat within 60 minutes after intense training and fuel workouts with protein plus slow carbohydrates.
2. **Schedule recovery like it's a performance strategy.**
   One to two full rest days weekly. A de-load week every 6–8 weeks. Muscle builds insulin sensitivity. Overtraining erodes it.
3. **Affirmation:**
   "Rest and nourishment amplify my power."

Why this works: The Achiever doesn't need more discipline. She needs metabolic safety.

The Survivor

Your Pattern: Survivors destabilize blood sugar through chronic stress history, emotional eating, or long-standing metabolic sluggishness.

Your Three Highest-Leverage Moves

1. **Anchor the day within 45 minutes of waking.**
   Protein-rich breakfast. Three meals spaced 3–4 hours apart. No grazing.
2. **Walk after meals.**
   Ten to fifteen minutes post-meal movement daily. Add strength training 2–3 times weekly to rebuild metabolic trust.
3. **Affirmation:**
   "I am safe in stability. My body is allowed to trust again."

Why this works: The Survivor's system needs rhythm, not extremes.

One Change—Today

Improving your health can feel overwhelming. With so many adjustments to make, habits to build, lab tests to do, results to interpret, supplements to add, even if you have a phenomenal healthcare team to support you, it can feel dizzying.

Remember that reversing the negative snowball and sending things in a positive direction begins with just *one step*.

Which of the three Hormone Types (Caretaker, Achiever, or Survivor) feels the closest to your current state? Knowing this, what is one small change you can make—today?

From Wild Swings to Stability

Remember Mia, the woman I introduced at the top of this chapter? The one who used to skip breakfast in the name of intermittent fasting? Who pushed her body to the limit with hardcore workouts and wasn't fueling herself enough to keep up with these demands?

After beginning her work with me, within three months, Mia's sugar cravings were gone, her afternoon energy crashes stopped, and she was finally sleeping through the night. Her cycles became regular again, her anxiety lifted, and her labs revealed levels in the optimal ranges. Her fasting insulin dropped, cortisol balanced out, and progesterone began to rise again with regular ovulation.

The secret wasn't another diet or detox. It was rhythm and stability. Her body just needed to be fed, rested, and trusted again.

Honestly, I get it. I've been there too.

As a Caretaker Type, I'm a former meal-skipper. I used to be the woman who bent over backwards to ensure that my daughters had a balanced, nutritious, protein-rich breakfast before school, and meanwhile, I was running on empty, with only coffee or matcha tea to fuel me. Back then, I thought being a good caregiver meant *sacrifice*—but now? I know that it means *role modeling*. How can I expect my daughters to take care of their incredible bodies if I am not leading by example?

I've learned that one of the most powerful things I can do for my hormones, my energy, and my sense of calm is to keep my blood sugar steady. When I eat breakfast before I caffeinate, anchor my meals with protein, work out to build muscle, and permit myself to rest instead of pushing through, everything changes. I think more clearly, feel more grounded and show up better for the people I love.

Balanced blood sugar isn't just about metabolism. It's about psychological safety. It's how we remind our bodies that we're not in survival mode, that it's safe to be alive, to flourish and thrive. When you feed yourself regularly and consistently, your body starts to trust you again. And that's where the deepest healing begins.

Key Takeaways

Balanced blood sugar = balanced hormones. When glucose levels are too high or too low, this can disrupt cortisol, estrogen, progesterone, and other hormones, leading to fatigue, anxiety, weight gain, and fertility challenges.

- Simple daily rhythms deliver big results. To stabilize your blood sugar naturally, these are the big five to remember:
  - Eat protein (20–30g) with every meal to slow down the release of glucose into your bloodstream.
  - Add fiber-rich foods to regulate glucose absorption.
  - Move for 10 minutes after meals. (And, add resistance training to your routine because stronger muscles reduce the risk of insulin resistance.)
  - Sleep between 10 p.m. to 6 a.m. to allow your body to rest and repair.
  - Practice stress-reducing rituals daily.
- Small, consistent steps like "breakfast before coffee" or "short walks after meals" compound into major improvements.
- Lab testing can illuminate blood sugar issues before they escalate into bigger problems, like insulin resistance or type 2 diabetes.
- Remember that just because lab testing shows a particular level within the normal range, "normal" and "optimal" are not the same thing.
- Supplements like chromium, magnesium, vitamin D, omega-3s, alpha-lipoic acid, and inositol—plus botanicals like cinnamon, fenugreek, and berberine—can support blood sugar stability. However, always check with your provider before using these, especially if you are already taking medication to manage your blood sugar.

- Steady is strong. Healing comes from establishing consistent rhythms, not perfection.
- Blood sugar balance isn't about restriction—like cutting out carbs or fasting until noon. It's about creating consistency in how you fuel, move, and rest. When your body senses steadiness, it feels safe and shifts from survival mode to thriving.

Notes

1. "Insulin Resistance of Puberty." Current Diabetes Reports. M. M. Kelsey & P. S. Zeitler. 2016. https://link.springer.com/article/10.1007/s11892-016-0751-5.
2. Kelsey, M. M., et al. (2020). The Impact of Obesity on Insulin Sensitivity and Secretion During Pubertal Progression: A Longitudinal Study. *The Journal of Clinical Endocrinology & Metabolism*. https://academic.oup.com/jcem/article/105/5/e2061/5717690.
3. "Longitudinal Predictors of Insulin Sensitivity and Secretion during Puberty." Diabetes. Authors not listed. 2018. https://diabetesjournals.org/diabetes/article/67/Supplement_1/1348-P/53954/Longitudinal-Predictors-of-Insulin-Sensitivity-and.
4. Waters, T. P., et al. (2019). Longitudinal Changes in Glucose Metabolism in Women with Gestational Diabetes, From Late Pregnancy to the Postpartum Period. https://link.springer.com/article/10.1007/s00125-019-05051-0.
5. Phaloprakarn, C., & Tangjitgamol, S. (2022). Glucose Levels during Gestational Diabetes Pregnancy and the Risk of Developing Postpartum Diabetes or Prediabetes. *BMC Pregnancy & Childbirth*. https://bmcpregnancychildbirth.biomedcentral.com/articles/10.1186/s12884-021-04352-w.
6. "Modifiable Risk Factors and Trends in Changes in Glucose Regulation During the First Three Years Postdelivery:

The St Carlos Gestational Diabetes Mellitus Prevention Cohort." Nutrients. Endocrinology and Nutrition Department, Hospital Clínico Universitario San Carlos, et al. 2023. https://www.mdpi.com/2072-6643/15/23/4995.

7. Bermingham, K. M., et al. (2022). Menopause Is Associated with Postprandial Metabolism, Metabolic Health and Lifestyle: The ZOE PREDICT Study. *eBioMedicine*. https://www.thelancet.com/journals/ebiom/article/PIIS2352-3964(22)00485-6/fulltext.
8. Zhu, J., et al. (2023). Role of Estrogen in the Regulation of Central and Peripheral Energy Homeostasis: From a Menopausal Perspective. *Therapeutic Advances in Endocrinology and Metabolism*. https://journals.sagepub.com/doi/10.1177/20420188231199359.
9. Bermingham, K., et al. (2022). Menopause Is a Key Factor Influencing Postprandial Metabolism, Metabolic Health and Lifestyle: The ZOE PREDICT Study. *Current Developments in Nutrition*. https://cdn.nutrition.org/article/S2475-2991(23)13020-4/pdf.
10. Tettamanzi, F., et al. (2021). A High Protein Diet Is More Effective in Improving Insulin Resistance and Glycemic Variability Compared to a Mediterranean Diet—A Cross-Over Controlled Inpatient Dietary Study. https://www.mdpi.com/2072-6643/13/12/4380.
11. Papakonstantinou, E., et al. (2022). Effects of Diet, Lifestyle, Chrononutrition and Alternative Dietary Interventions on Postprandial Glycemia and Insulin Resistance. https://www.mdpi.com/2072-6643/14/4/823.
12. Basciani, S., et al. (2025). Unexpected Effects of Treating Insulin-Resistant Obese Women with High-Dose D-chiro-inositol: Opening Pandora's Box. https://www.frontiersin.org/journals/endocrinology/articles/10.3389/fendo.2025.1399308/full.

13. Samiilenko, N., et al. (2024). Gender-Specific Effects of 3-Month Nutrition Intervention on Lipid Profiles and Insulin Sensitivity. *Proceedings of the Nutrition Society*. https://www.cambridge.org/core/journals/proceedings-of-the-nutrition-society/article/genderspecific-effects-of-3month-nutrition-intervention-on-lipid-profiles-and-insulin-sensitivity/AC8FED050FA39F2F7EC218CE3017A448.
14. Murugesan, R., et al. (2024). Food Order Affects Blood Glucose and Insulin Levels in Women with Gestational Diabetes. *Frontiers in Nutrition*. https://www.frontiersin.org/journals/nutrition/articles/10.3389/fnut.2024.1512231/full.
15. Zhang, L., et al. (2024). Effects of Dietary Approaches and Exercise Interventions on Gestational Diabetes Mellitus: A Systematic Review and Bayesian Network Meta-Analysis. https://www.sciencedirect.com/science/article/pii/S2161831324001649?via%3Dihub.
16. Jin, S., et al. (2020). Effects of Nutritional Strategies on Glucose Homeostasis in Gestational Diabetes Mellitus: A Systematic Review and Network Meta-Analysis. https://onlinelibrary.wiley.com/doi/10.1155/2020/6062478.
17. "The Benefits of Seed Cycling." Dr. Corina Dunlap. 2022. https://drcorinadunlap.com/the-benefits-of-seed-cycling/.
18. "Beeya Clinical Study: Detailed Report." *Beeya Wellness*. Beeya Wellness. 2025. cdn.shopify.com/s/files/1/0514/1102/6118/files/Beeya_Clinical_Study_-_Detailed_Report.pdf.
19. "Short Walks After Meals Deliver Big Benefits for Blood Glucose." News-Medical. Pramanik, P. 2025. https://www.news-medical.net/news/20250703/Short-walks-after-meals-deliver-big-benefits-for-blood-glucose.
20. "A 10-Minute Walk After a Meal 'Good for Diabetes'." NICSwell. 2025. https://www.nicswell.co.uk/health-news/a-10-minute-walk-after-a-meal-good-for-diabetes.

21. Xie, Y., et al. (2020). A Meta-Analysis of the Effects of Resistance Training on Blood Sugar and Pregnancy Outcomes https://www.sciencedirect.com/science/article/pii/S0266613820302114?via%3Dihub.
22. "Abstract P437: Early Insulin Resistance Responds to Lifestyle Interventions: The Premier Study." *Circulation*, American Heart Association. Cistola, D. P., et al. 2020. https://www.ahajournals.org/doi/10.1161/circ.141.suppl_1.P437.
23. Guo, J., et al. (2016). Postpartum Lifestyle Interventions to Prevent type 2 Diabetes Among Women with History of Gestational Diabetes: A Systematic Review of Randomized Clinical Trials. *Journal of Women's Health*. https://www.liebertpub.com/doi/10.1089/jwh.2015.5262.
24. Papakonstantinou, E., et al. (2022). Effects of Diet, Lifestyle, Chrononutrition and Alternative Dietary Interventions on Postprandial Glycemia and Insulin Resistance. *Nutrients*. https://www.mdpi.com/2072-6643/14/4/823.
25. "Preventing Muscle Loss as We Age." Ohio State Health & Discovery. Vavrek, K. 2024. https://health.osu.edu/wellness/exercise-and-nutrition/preventing-muscle-loss-as-we-age#.
26. "The Many Benefits of Resistance Training as You Age." Mayo Clinic Press. Bowman, A. 2024. https://mcpress.mayoclinic.org/healthy-aging/the-many-benefits-of-resistance-training-as-you-age/#.
27. Basciani, S., et al. (2025). Unexpected Effects of Treating Insulin-Resistant Obese Women with High-Dose D-chiro-inositol: Opening Pandora's Box. https://www.frontiersin.org/journals/endocrinology/articles/10.3389/fendo.2025.1399308/full.
28. Samiilenko, N., et al. (2024). Gender-Specific Effects of 3-month Nutrition Intervention on Lipid Profiles and Insulin Sensitivity. *Proceedings of the Nutrition Society*. https://www.cam

bridge.org/core/journals/proceedings-of-the-nutrition-society/article/genderspecific-effects-of-3month-nutrition-intervention-on-lipid-profiles-and-insulin-sensitivity/AC8FED050FA39F2F7EC218CE3017A448.

29. Papakonstantinou, E., et al. (2022). Effects of Diet, Lifestyle, Chrononutrition and Alternative Dietary Interventions on Postprandial Glycemia and Insulin Resistance. https://www.mdpi.com/2072-6643/14/4/823.

Chapter 8

Get Deep, Restorative Sleep

When my daughters were three years old and nine months old, I entered an exceptionally demanding season of my life and career. We had recently relocated from Oregon to Maine, where I opened my new practice and was busily building my client roster in a new state. On top of that, I was flying back to the West Coast twice a month to teach medical students at a graduate school where I served as an adjunct professor and saw patients at my old clinic there. All while raising a toddler, nursing an infant, being woken up multiple times a night for feedings, and going through the postpartum roller coaster, for the second time in three years.

Although I tend to have an optimistic outlook ("I got this. I'm powerful and strong. I chose this life, and I can handle it. Everything is going to work out. . ."), over time, this schedule wore me down. The constant flights. Time zone changes. Jet lag. Disrupted sleep. Not to mention the stress of squeezing in time to pump milk six times a day (practically a full-time job) when I was at the clinic with my patients or on a work trip, although I had a supportive husband, and in-laws who were willing to help out with childcare, my village wasn't enough to counteract the mounting exhaustion I felt. Eventually, I reached my breaking point.

I remember rushing to catch a flight, feeling frantic, on the verge of a panic attack, with an overwhelming sense of "something is not right" and "I can't do this anymore" building up inside my body. I was worn out in a way I had never experienced before. It was more than the temporary fatigue that mothers with babies often feel from 2 a.m. night feedings. It was deeper than that.

That's when I admitted to myself, "Although I have dedicated my career to helping women achieve optimal health, the patient who needs the most attention right now is *me*." I was stretching myself to the brink, caring for others—my family, my patients, my students—without giving my body the rest it needed to keep up with all the demands.

To bring myself back into balance, I created my own personal Hormone Action Plan, with a strong focus on deep, restorative sleep. Because when you're not sleeping well, to quote Marjorie Soltis, MD, "It literally makes every other component of our life and health worse. It makes pain worse, it makes anxiety worse, it makes depression worse."

Author JoJo Jensen adds to the conversation, saying, "Without enough sleep, we all become tall two-year-olds." She's right. When sleep-deprived, we struggle with everything from emotional regulation and impulse control to planning and problem-solving and beyond.

But what many of my clients don't realize is that it's not just the *amount* of sleep you're getting that matters. It's also the *quality* of your sleep that determines if your body is truly getting the recovery and regeneration time that it needs.

Sleep: The Medicine We Overlook

Sleep might be one of my favorite topics as a doctor, a mom, and a woman. Over the years, I've come to see sleep as one of the most potent health levers we have. It affects not only how long we live, but how well we live. Sleep influences every system in the body and shapes how we feel in every decade of life.

Through research, through the stories of my patients, and through my own life, I've witnessed how transformational quality sleep can be. I've also seen how quickly life unravels when it's missing. When we protect sleep, we protect everything it touches: hormone balance, fertility, metabolism, immunity, mood, and even our long-term risk of chronic disease. Few things matter more.

Sleep isn't just rest. It's active repair. It's hormonal recalibration. It's emotional and physical detox. And it is one of the greatest gifts you can give yourself at any stage of life. As I move through the decades, I've become more devoted to my sleep routine and far less willing to compromise it. Once you've experienced the clarity, vitality, and steadiness that come from deep rest, you stop seeing it as optional.

Writing this chapter feels like offering a gift. It's a love letter to women everywhere and to our daughters and granddaughters who deserve to know what real rest feels like.

Sleep is essential for everyone, yet women face unique challenges. Hormonal fluctuations across the month and across the lifespan profoundly influence sleep architecture and circadian rhythm. Layered on top of that, women also have sleep challenges due to demanding careers, raising children, and all the other roles we play in our families and communities. Most women who come to our clinic struggle with some form of disordered sleep. Many sense that hormones are involved, and they're not wrong. What they may not realize, however, is how cyclical the relationship truly is. Hormonal imbalance can disrupt sleep, and poor sleep deepens hormonal imbalance.

This chapter is about breaking that cycle.

How Are You Sleeping?

When I meet a new patient, I often start with five simple questions:

- How many hours of sleep are you getting?
- What time do you fall asleep?
- Do you wake up during the night?
- Do you dream?
- Do you wake up feeling rested?

I pay close attention to how women answer these questions. Their tone, their body language, and the emotions that surface tell me just as much as their words. Many women already know how essential sleep is, yet over time they've learned to normalize their exhaustion. Some even wear it like a badge of honor, a sign of "caring about others" or "working hard to achieve important goals." Others have convinced themselves that they are "just night owls" or that needing less sleep is simply how they're wired.

These questions—and a woman's answers—reveal far more than bedtime habits. They show me how the woman's body is regenerating (or not), how steady her nervous system feels, and how well her hormones are communicating. Because sleep isn't just the absence of wakefulness. It's the foundation of hormone health itself.

What Is Deep, Restorative Sleep?

Deep, restorative sleep is when your body does its most important overnight work: cellular repair, hormone rebalancing, immune regulation, and nervous system reset. This doesn't just depend on how many hours you're in bed; it's all about sleep architecture.

Sleep architecture[1] refers to how you move through the different stages of sleep. There are four stages of sleep. The first three are non-rapid eye movement stages, and the fourth includes rapid-eye movement. In a nutshell, the four sleep phases go like this. . .

Stage 1: Light Sleep

In this phase, you're transitioning from wakefulness to sleep. Your heartbeat, breathing, and eye movements slow down, and your muscles relax. It's fairly easy to wake someone up when they're in the light sleep phase. This phase generally lasts a short amount of time. It's the transitional portal into rest.

Stage 2: True Sleep

Your heart rate and breathing continue to slow down, you become unaware of your surroundings, and it is harder to wake up. This phase is longer than its predecessor, light sleep. During the N2 stage, your brain activity shifts, beginning to show the signs of slow-wave brain activity, otherwise known as delta waves.

Stage 3: Slow-Wave Sleep

This is the deepest stage of sleep. Your brain activity has shifted fully into delta waves. If you were hooked up to a scanning device monitoring the electrical activity in your brain, the imagery on the screen would look like long, slow, gently rolling waves.

Slow-wave sleep is critical for the body's repair system—this is when growth hormone is released, helping rebuild tissues and muscles. This phase of sleep enhances the immune system and promotes the production of cytokines, which fight infection and reduce inflammation. And the delta waves that occur during deep sleep are like a cleansing shampoo for your brain cells. Delta waves help activate the glymphatic system, which clears out waste products like amyloid plaques (clumps of protein) that build up in your brain during the day.

Stage 4: Rapid Eye Movement (REM) Sleep

After slow-wave sleep comes REM sleep. This is where your brain resets. REM sleep supports memory consolidation, learning, creativity, and emotional processing. During this stage, your eyes move rapidly behind your eyelids. Brain activity shifts closer to wakefulness—those long, slow, rolling brain waves become shorter and faster. Most vivid dreaming occurs during this stage. Neurochemicals like GABA and glycine keep your voluntary muscles (like your arms and legs) in a state of temporary paralysis, a natural protective measure to keep you from acting out your dreams.

For adults, it takes about 90–110 minutes to go through an entire sleep cycle—this means progressing through all four stages: light, true, slow-wave, and REM. During a good night's sleep, you'll have four to six complete cycles, which allows your body and brain to function at their best.

The final two stages of the sleep cycle—slow-wave sleep and REM sleep—are what I call **deep, restorative sleep**. These stages are when deep regeneration, deep cleansing, and deep healing happens.

Slow-wave and REM are the two heavy-hitters when it comes to hormonal health. When these stages aren't happening like they should, this means you're getting "some" sleep but not the deep, restorative kind. You feel it—in the form of brain fog, lethargy, low mood, and other indicators of poor-quality sleep. You could be getting plenty of sleep, in terms of the number of hours, but if you're not getting enough slow-wave and REM time, then you wake up and still don't feel rested.

The VIHs of Sleep

Remember in Chapter 1 when we introduced the very important hormones (VIHs)? These same hormones are deeply intertwined with sleep. In fact, research shows a direct relationship between these key hormones and the quality of your sleep. Think of hormones as the conductors of your sleep symphony: they cue your brain when to be alert, when to wind down, when to repair, and how to balance stress, sex, and rest. So let's reintroduce the VIHs of the female hormone world and explore how they shape your sleep.

Melatonin: The Master Clock Setter

Melatonin is produced by the pineal gland in response to darkness. It tells your body, "It's nighttime," and aligns your circadian rhythm, your 24-hour biological clock.

It helps synchronize the HPA (stress axis) and HPG (reproductive axis).

It acts like a gentle switch, helping you fall asleep but also setting the timing for hormonal events overnight.

Progesterone: The Natural Sedative

Often called the body's "chill pill," progesterone activates GABA receptors, which have calming effects on the brain.

High progesterone (like in the luteal phase or pregnancy) can enhance deep sleep.

Low progesterone (like when we don't ovulate and in perimenopause/menopause) is linked to more sleep disturbances and anxiety.

Estrogen: The Thermostat and REM Regulator

Estrogen plays a key role in thermoregulation and REM sleep modulation.

It keeps body temperature stable, which is crucial for staying asleep.

It promotes more time in REM sleep, the phase needed for learning and mood stability.

Testosterone: The Rebuilder

While often associated with men, testosterone is essential for women too, especially for energy, mood, and muscle recovery.

Testosterone levels rise during deep sleep, supporting muscle repair and tissue regeneration.

Poor sleep disrupts testosterone production, which can reduce libido, energy, and overall vitality.

Cortisol: The Rhythmic Alarm Clock

Cortisol is your body's main stress hormone and has a clear daily rhythm that should look like this:

Peak upon waking known as the *cortisol awakening response* (CAR). It helps you feel alert and ready to take on the day.
Steady decline through the day maintaining focus and energy.
Low at bedtime allowing melatonin to rise and sleep to begin.
Lowest during the night, so your body can repair without interference from stress signals.

When cortisol is too high at night (often due to stress or circadian disruption), it blocks melatonin, delays sleep, and fragments your deep stages, especially slow-wave and REM.

This chart gives a quick summary of what happens during the deep, restorative sleep phases—that's slow-wave sleep and REM sleep—sleep stages and hormonal benefits.

Reflect

Answer these five sleep questions that I ask my patients:

1. How many hours of sleep are you getting?
2. What time do you fall asleep?
3. Do you wake up during the night?
4. Do you dream?
5. And do you wake up feeling rested?

Here are the ideal answers: 7–9 hours, before 10 p.m., not often, yes, and yes.

If your answers are different, that's a sign that your sleep routine needs a tune-up. It's likely that you're not getting enough slow-wave and REM sleep.

Do Men and Women Sleep Differently?

Yes, and the science is clear: biological sex influences sleep needs, patterns, and quality.

Women:

- Tend to have more slow-wave sleep than men, which is generally beneficial for physical and cognitive repair.
- Are more prone to insomnia, especially during hormonal transitions (e.g., luteal phase, perimenopause, menopause).
- Experience more frequent sleep fragmentation due to hormonal fluctuations in estrogen and progesterone.
- May have longer total sleep durations but report poorer sleep quality, particularly during the luteal phase and perimenopause/menopause.

Men:

- Have higher levels of testosterone, which depend heavily on deep sleep for overnight replenishment.
- They are more likely to experience sleep apnea and other breathing-related sleep disorders, often linked to physical differences in airway structure and body composition.
- May enter REM sleep more quickly but spend slightly less time in deep sleep compared to women.

Why It Matters

These differences mean women may need slightly more sleep overall and may benefit more from routines that support hormonal stability and settling the nervous system. Men, on the other hand, may need strategies to optimize testosterone recovery and breathing efficiency.

While the foundation of an ideal sleep pattern is similar for men and women, women generally have longer and objectively higher-quality sleep but are more prone to sleep complaints and insomnia, especially during hormonal transitions like pregnancy, postpartum, perimenopause, and menopause. Men are more affected by sleep apnea and may have more fragmented sleep with age. Tailoring sleep recommendations to account for these differences can help optimize sleep health for both sexes.

Dreaming: The Brain's Emotional Editing Suite

Why do we dream? Dreaming is one of the most fascinating and essential functions of the human brain. During REM sleep, your mind works through the events and emotions of your waking life, helping you process experiences, reduce stress, and regulate mood. This is the stage where memory consolidation happens: your brain reviews what it learned, decides what to keep, and files it away for later. Dreams also open the door to creativity. When the logical parts of the brain quiet down, the imagination begins to connect ideas that would never meet in the light of day, often leading to fresh insights and breakthroughs. Research even shows that people who dream about a problem are more likely to find a solution to it the next day.

Dreams occur during REM sleep, the fourth part of the sleep cycle, which becomes longer and more vivid in the second half of the night. This is one reason staying asleep until morning is so important. If you regularly wake up too early, you may be missing out on your richest and most restorative dream cycles.

Dreaming is one of the few brain activities that completely ignores external reality. It's your mind's private sandbox, a nightly world of repair, imagination, and meaning that plays a vital role in your emotional and mental health.

The Hormonal Cost of Poor Sleep

When you're not getting enough sleep—particularly slow-wave sleep and REM sleep, which is when deep restoration occurs—what happens on a hormonal level?

Cortisol Dysregulation

- Poor sleep increases evening cortisol levels, a stress hormone, which can elevate anxiety and promote fat storage, especially in the abdominal area.[2]
- Higher cortisol during sleep deprivation correlates with impaired glucose regulation.[3]
- Cortisol also modulates REM and slow-wave sleep, further affecting sleep quality.[4]

Insulin Resistance

- Even short-term sleep restriction significantly reduces insulin sensitivity and contributes to hyperglycemia.[5]
- Sleep loss impairs metabolic function, increasing the risk of type 2 diabetes.[6]
- Sleep restriction is associated with elevated fasting glucose and disrupted glucose tolerance.[7]

Leptin and Ghrelin Imbalance

- Sleep loss lowers leptin (which suppresses appetite) and increases ghrelin (which promotes hunger), leading to increased food cravings and risk of obesity.[8]
- Ghrelin also boosts cortisol and growth hormone when administered early in the morning, reflecting its strong influence on metabolic hormones.[9]

Reproductive Hormone Disruption, Diminished Ovarian Reserve, and Fertility Implications

- Sleep loss is associated with reduced testosterone and other anabolic hormones, impacting fertility and reproductive health.[10]
- Sleep loss is increasingly recognized as a modifiable risk factor for diminished ovarian reserve and possibly poorer egg quality, especially in women over 35 or those already facing fertility challenges. Improving sleep hygiene can play a supportive role in protecting reproductive potential.[11,12]

Thyroid Suppression

- Poor sleep increases TSH and active thyroid hormones (like T3), leading to sluggish metabolism and low energy, more hypothyroid symptoms.[13]
- Poor sleep is associated with a higher risk of thyroid dysfunction and can negatively influence thyroid health in women.

The takeaway? Deep, restorative sleep is your nightly opportunity to reset every major system in the body and is one of the most massive keys to reaching your hormone power. Prioritize sleep quality, honor your body's natural rhythms, and you'll begin to feel the difference in your mind, mood, metabolism, and overall quality of life.

So, how can you start getting higher-quality sleep? Next, I'll present an ideal sleep plan for women.

> **Reflect**
>
> When was the last time you woke up feeling truly rested? What changes in your life might be stealing your sleep without you realizing it?

An Ideal Nightly Sleep Pattern for Women

If you began getting the highest-quality sleep of your life tonight, what would it look like?

Research is remarkably consistent.

- 7–9 hours per night
- Asleep before 10 p.m. when possible
- Minimal awakenings
- Consistent sleep and wake times, even on weekends
- Protection of the 10 p.m. to 6 a.m. hormonal repair window

Duration matters. But quality matters just as much.[14,15]

High-quality sleep means moving through full sleep cycles, including slow-wave sleep and REM sleep. This is when growth hormone is released, memories consolidate, cortisol recalibrates, and emotional tone stabilizes.[16]

Sleep timing also matters. Earlier bedtimes are consistently associated with better metabolic and mental health outcomes in women. Large swings between weekday and weekend schedules, often called "social jet lag," disrupt circadian rhythm and increase stress hormone activation.

As women move through different life stages, sleep architecture may shift slightly. But the foundational recommendation remains the same: protect your hours, protect your rhythm, protect your darkness.[17]

Sleep Stealers and Sleep Supporters

Why does it feel so hard to get a good night's sleep? Multiple lifestyle factors have been shown to impact sleep quality in women. I call these "sleep stealers." The sneaky thieves that rob you of deep, restorative sleep. These influences are often interrelated and can vary across life stages.

The Sleep Stealers

Sedentary living

Long stretches of sitting blunt circadian signaling and reduce sleep drive. Daily movement, especially earlier in the day, strengthens sleep architecture.[18,19]

Late-night eating and unstable blood sugar

Heavy meals close to bedtime raise insulin and suppress melatonin. Blood sugar drops at 2–3 a.m. can trigger cortisol spikes and wakefulness.[20,21]

Excess screen exposure
Blue light in the evening delays melatonin release and keeps your brain in "daytime mode."[22]

Caffeine and alcohol
Caffeine lingers longer than most women realize. Alcohol may make you sleepy initially but fragments deep sleep later in the night.[23,24]

Chronic stress
Elevated evening cortisol blocks melatonin and reduces slow-wave and REM sleep.[25]

Environmental factors
Having a poor sleep environment (it's too noisy, too bright, too hot, too cold, or your bed is uncomfortable) can worsen sleep quality. Sleeping with noise in the background—such as music, a podcast, or the TV on—is a definite sleep stealer.[26]

Hormonal transitions
Perimenopause, postpartum shifts, thyroid changes, and metabolic instability all influence sleep architecture.

The Sleep Supporters Good sleep starts the moment you wake up.

Think of every part of your day (light, movement, food, screen time) as cues that set the rhythm for your brain and body. You're not just trying to fall asleep at bedtime—you're training your internal clock to stay aligned with the natural world, and the benefits extend to mood, metabolism, hormone balance, immune function, and cognitive clarity.

Here are the highest-leverage lifestyle sleep supporters.

Sync with Light

- Morning light within 30–60 minutes of waking.
  Step outside. Even cloudy light works. This anchors cortisol and sets melatonin timing 14–16 hours later.

- Dim lights after sunset.
  Lower overhead lighting. Reduce screen use 1–2 hours before bed. Think warm, soft, quiet. Your pineal gland responds to darkness. Protect it.

A note about the best type of light exposure for circadian support after sunset:

- Even low levels of artificial light at night (as little as 10–30 lux) can suppress melatonin and delay your body clock.
- Blue light (460–480 nm)—common in screens and indoor lighting—is especially disruptive to sleep and circadian rhythms.
- Red or warm light (606–635 nm) is much less disruptive and may even counteract the effects of blue light. If you absolutely must look at a screen after sundown, switch to "night mode," which generally emits a warm yellow glow.

Time Your Meals

- Eat within 1 hour of waking to anchor your body clock.
- Avoid large meals 2–3 hours before bed to prevent insulin-related disruption of melatonin.

Eat for Sleep

- Avoid caffeine after 12 to 2 p.m., and limit or avoid alcohol altogether, as it fragments deep sleep.
- Balanced protein and complex carbohydrates at dinner can support serotonin and melatonin production.
- Magnesium-rich foods (like leafy greens, pumpkin seeds, and avocado) support relaxation and melatonin production.

Support Temperature

- Aim for cool room temps (65–68°F) at bedtime to mimic nighttime environmental signals.
- A warm shower or bath 60–90 minutes before bed helps drop core body temperature, triggering melatonin release.

Create a Wind-Down Ritual

- Power down devices or use blue light filters 1 to 2 hours before bed.
- Consider a "tech curfew" or "digital sundown" and swap screens for journaling, light reading, or gentle stretching.

Make Your Bedroom a Sanctuary

- Make your bedroom pitch dark. You shouldn't be able to see your hand in front of your face.
- Use blackout curtains, cover LEDs, remove glowing electronics, or, better yet, turn them off.
- Power down wireless Internet to limit EMF nighttime exposure in the home.

Long-Term Rewiring

To achieve high-quality sleep, your goal is to minimize *sleep stealers* and use more *sleep supporters*. Doing this will change the way you sleep. You may wake up tomorrow feeling more rested than you have felt in a long time!

However, think of this as nervous system retraining—not a quick fix. Getting deep, restorative sleep requires more than just being "tired enough" at bedtime. It's about sending consistent signals to your body throughout the day that guide you into rest-and-repair mode. With time, this becomes effortless, like tuning your body back into its natural rhythm.

Reflect

What is one sleep stealer that you can eliminate from your life, effective immediately?

What is one sleep supporter you can add in?

Botanicals and Targeted Sleep Support

If foundational supports are in place and sleep still feels fragile, targeted support can help. Start simple and layer intentionally. More is not necessarily better. In practice, I find there is not a one-size-fits-all approach. These must be individualized. Rather than combining multiple herbs at once, begin with one and assess response over one to two weeks.

Evidence-Supported Botanicals

Valerian root (Valeriana officinalis)[27]
May reduce sleep latency and improve sleep quality through GABA modulation. Best for difficulty falling asleep.

Lavender (Lavandula)[28]
Supports relaxation and reduces nighttime anxiety. Helpful for stress-driven insomnia.

Passionflower (Passiflora incarnata)[29]
Gentle calming herb that supports nervous system downshifting, especially when thoughts are looping at night.

Chamomile (Matricaria recutita)[30]
Mild sedative properties. Useful for light, fragmented sleep.

Lemon Balm (Melissa officinalis) and California Poppy (Eschscholzia californica)[31]
Some evidence for sleep promotion.

Magnolia (Magnolia officinalis)[32]
Supports GABA and serotonin pathways. Particularly helpful during postpartum or perimenopausal transitions.

Non-Botanical Support

Melatonin[33,34,35]

Melatonin supplementation is well tolerated and effective for improving sleep onset, duration, and quality, especially in circadian rhythm disorders and in older adults. Melatonin is considered safe and non-habit-forming, with most side effects being mild and short-lived (for example: fatigue, vivid dreams). Typical doses range from 0.3 to 3 milligrams taken 30–60 minutes before bed, though smaller doses often work best and more closely mimic the body's natural rhythm.

Like vitamin D, melatonin has become one of the modern world's hidden deficiencies, largely due to our constant exposure to artificial light. Reestablishing a healthy relationship with light and darkness may be one of the most powerful ways to reclaim deep, restorative sleep. Still, melatonin is often added and is especially helpful for women in hormonal transitions.

As women age, melatonin production tends to decline, and this drop can be worsened by stress, late-night light exposure, endometriosis, or menopausal hormone shifts. Supplementing can be especially helpful for restoring sleep during these transitions.

Magnesium (glycinate or L-threonate)[36,37]

Supports relaxation and may improve sleep efficiency. Particularly helpful in women with stress-driven tension. Magnesium-L-threonate (MgT) has superior brain bioavailability and is the most well-researched for sleep quality.

L-theanine[38]

Reduces sleep latency and supports calm mental states without sedation.

Glycine[39]

Can support sleep onset and quality, especially when core body temperature regulation is disrupted.

Phosphatidylserine[40]

Useful when elevated evening cortisol is preventing sleep onset.

Doing Everything Right—But Still Tired?

Doing your daily nervous system hygiene? Check. Keep your blood sugar stable? Check. Minimizing sleep stealers and using sleep supporters? Check and check.

If you feel like you're "doing everything right," yet your sleep still feels disrupted or not as refreshing as you'd hope, lab testing can help uncover what's driving it beneath the surface.

Sleep challenges are rarely just about sleep itself—they often reflect hormonal, metabolic, or nervous system imbalances that can be identified and corrected with the right testing.

Here are the most strategic labs to consider in collaboration with your provider.

Which Tests to Do

Cortisol + Adrenal Rhythm

A four-point cortisol test (saliva, serum, or urine) maps your stress rhythm.

We're looking for:

- Elevated evening cortisol
- Flattened daily curve
- Low morning peak

All of these can fragment slow-wave and REM sleep.

Thyroid Panel

TSH, Free T4, Free T3 ± antibodies.

Even mild thyroid dysfunction can impair temperature regulation, metabolism, and sleep quality.

Sex Hormones

- Estradiol + FSH/LH: ideally tested Days 2–5
- Progesterone: 5–7 days post-ovulation
- Testosterone + SHBG: any cycle day

Low progesterone, fluctuating estrogen, or declining ovarian reserve can contribute to insomnia, night sweats, and early waking.

Iron + Ferritin

Low ferritin (especially below 50 ng/mL) is a common and overlooked cause of restless sleep and nighttime awakenings.

Glucose + Insulin
Fasting glucose, HbA1c, and fasting insulin.

Nocturnal hypoglycemia or insulin resistance can trigger 2–4 a.m. cortisol spikes.

Foundational Nutrients
Vitamin D, RBC magnesium, B12.

These nutrients support neurotransmitter production and circadian signaling.

When to Consider a Sleep Study
If you snore, wake gasping, or never feel restored despite adequate hours, evaluate for sleep apnea. Repeated oxygen dips fragment deep sleep and elevate cortisol over time.

What We're Looking For
Patterns—not just isolated numbers.

- High evening cortisol
- Low progesterone
- Elevated FSH in perimenopause or those with suspected POI
- Suboptimal thyroid conversion
- Low ferritin
- Rising fasting insulin

Once the driver is identified, treatment becomes precise.

Rest Goes Beyond Sleep

You're following all the best practices for deep, restorative sleep. You're getting seven to nine hours every night. Your labs are looking good. Things are moving in the right direction. Yet, despite all this effort, you *still* don't feel well-rested. What's going on?

Dr. Saundra Dalton-Smith, board-certified internal medicine physician and author of *Sacred Rest*,[41] noticed this happening frequently with her patients. Women often told her, "I'm getting deep sleep, yet I feel tired...." It is almost as if there's a tank that's empty that no amount of sleep can fill.

This prompted Dr. Dalton-Smith to get curious about what it means to be "exhausted" and what it means to "recharge," not just from a purely physical level but on a spiritual level as well.

As Dr. Dalton-Smith explains in her book, if you're already getting high-quality sleep, then "more sleep" isn't necessarily going to make you feel "more rested."You may need a different form of rest instead—the kind that happens when you are awake.

For example, if you are *emotionally* exhausted from a messy divorce, you may need the restoration that comes from a walk with a friend, therapy, creative self-expression, or a good cry. If you are experiencing *social* exhaustion from a jam-packed calendar, you may need the kind of rest that comes from stillness and silence. If you're dealing with *sensory* exhaustion from too much screen time or over-exposure to bright lights and loud noises, the rest you need might be found in a long hike in the woods or a no-tech weekend. Being alone, being with others, music, movement, connection with your inner wisdom or a higher power, experiencing a moment of sublime beauty or awe—all of these can be powerful forms of rest, too.

If you are doing everything right when it comes to sleep but still feel tired, consider, "Is there another form of rest that I need—beyond sleep?" Rest, says Dr. Dalton-Smith, comes in many forms, and it is "something sacred, valuable, and worthy of our respect."

Reflect

In addition to high-quality sleep, what's another form of rest that you need right now?

It could be the restoration that comes from laughter, time in nature, or an afternoon with zero responsibilities.

Specific Recommendations for the Caretaker, Achiever, and Survivor

Sleep is one of the most powerful hormone therapies available. Whether you're a Caretaker, Achiever, or Survivor, you need seven to nine hours of high-quality sleep, circadian rhythm support through light exposure, consistent meal timing, and evening wind-down rituals. But, depending on whether you're a Caretaker, Achiever, or Survivor, you can focus your approach to align with your Hormone Type. Here are my recommendations.

The Caretaker

Your Pattern: Caretakers destabilize sleep by staying up too late for everyone else and under-fueling their own nervous system.

Your Three Highest-Leverage Moves

1. **Eat a protein-forward dinner before 7 p.m.**
   Stable blood sugar overnight prevents 2–3 a.m. cortisol spikes and anxious wake-ups.
2. **Create a hard "digital sunset."**
   Lights down and screens off at least 60 minutes before bed. The world can wait. Your nervous system cannot.
3. **Affirmation:**
   "Resting refills my capacity to care."

Why this works: The Caretaker's insomnia is usually depletion-driven. Stability and boundaries restore sleep depth.

The Achiever

Your Pattern: Achievers destabilize sleep through overstimulation and elevated evening cortisol. The body is tired. The mind is not.

Your Three Highest-Leverage Moves

1. **Protect a 90-minute wind-down window.**
   No work, no planning, no productivity. Journal tomorrow's tasks so your brain doesn't rehearse them at 1 a.m.

2. **Lower evening cortisol intentionally.**
   Gentle breathwork, magnesium, or phosphatidylserine at dinner can help shift from performance mode to repair mode.
3. **Affirmation:**
   "My rest is the most productive thing I do."

Why this works: The Achiever doesn't need more discipline. She needs permission to downshift.

The Survivor

Your Pattern: Survivors often struggle with light, fragmented sleep due to chronic stress imprinting on the nervous system.

Your Three Highest-Leverage Moves

1. **Anchor morning light within 30 minutes of waking.**
   This strengthens circadian rhythm and reduces nighttime cortisol activation.
2. **Create a safety cue at bedtime.**
   Cool, dark, quiet room. Weighted blanket, white noise, or grounding ritual to calm hypervigilance.
3. **Affirmation:**
   "My body is safe to rest now."

Why this works: The Survivor's sleep improves when the nervous system feels secure, not stimulated.

Sleep Is Shaped by Every Choice

There are many things in this world that we can't control. But one thing we have a great deal of power and agency over is our sleep. What time you begin your caffeine curfew, what time you have dinner and what you eat, when you turn off the devices—all of these are largely within your control.

Remember that deep, restorative sleep begins in the morning, and the choices you make all day long will either support your sleep—or steal from it.

Remember, too, that optimal health isn't about "perfection." If you have a late-night sugary snack or curl up with your iPad to watch your favorite TV show until 10 p.m. occasionally, this won't derail your health. But what are you doing most nights? Most days? Most of the time? Make sure that your standard routine includes plenty of sleep supporters and minimal sleep stealers. That's how you'll wake up revitalized, feeling like your most powerful self.

Key Takeaways

- *Deep, restorative sleep isn't passive*—it's active repair. This is when your body resets hormonal balance, repairs tissues, cleanses debris from your brain, and restores emotional equilibrium.
- *Quality, not just quantity.* You need seven to nine hours of high-quality sleep each night. This means moving through the full sleep cycle, particularly the slow-wave phase and REM phase, when deep restoration occurs.
- *Great sleep begins in the morning.* Waking up with the sun, physical movement throughout the day, reducing screen time and light exposure after sundown—all of your daily decisions either support or sabotage your sleep.
- *There's more to rest than just sleep.* Exhaustion isn't always cured by getting more sleep. Emotional, mental, creative, and spiritual rest are equally vital forms of recovery, too. Identify what kind of rest you truly need—connection, solitude, beauty, stillness—and honor it as sacred.

- *Start with one step.* Could you try a caffeine curfew earlier in the day? Wind down for bedtime with a journal instead of your phone? Put blackout curtains in your bedroom? Make one adjustment today, and another tomorrow, and watch the impact stack up.

Notes

1. Fattinger, S., et al. (2017). Deep Sleep Maintains Learning Efficiency of the Human Brain. *Nature Communications*. https://www.nature.com/articles/ncomms15405.
2. Giannos, P., et al. (2023). Shorter Sleep Duration Is Associated with Greater Visceral Fat Mass in US Adults: Findings from NHANES, 2011–2014. https://www.sciencedirect.com/science/article/pii/S1389945723000990?via%3Dihub.
3. AlDabal, L., & BaHammam, A. S. (2011). Metabolic, Endocrine, and Immune Consequences of Sleep Deprivation. *Open Respiratory Medicine Journal*. http://openrespiratorymedicinejournal.com/VOLUME/05/PAGE/31/.
4. Born, J. (2004). Memory Consolidation During Sleep: Role of Cortisol Feedback. *Annals of the New York Academy of Sciences*. 7. https://nyaspubs.onlinelibrary.wiley.com/doi/10.1196/annals.1314.020.
5. Broussard, J. L., et al. (2012). Impaired Insulin Signaling in Human Adipocytes After Experimental Sleep Restriction: A Randomized, Crossover Study. https://www.acpjournals.org/doi/10.7326/0003-4819-157-8-201210160-00005.
6. Briançon-Marjollet, A., et al. (2015). The Impact of Sleep Disorders on Glucose Metabolism: Endocrine and Molecular Mechanisms. *Diabetology & Metabolic Syndrome*. https://dmsjournal.biomedcentral.com/articles/10.1186/s13098-015-0018-3.

7. Gottlieb, D. J., et al. (2005). Association of Sleep Time with Diabetes Mellitus and Impaired Glucose Tolerance. *Archives of Internal Medicine.* https://jamanetwork.com/journals/jamainternalmedicine/fullarticle/486518.
8. Taheri, S., et al. (2004). Short Sleep Duration Is Associated with Reduced Leptin, Elevated Ghrelin, and Increased Body Mass Index. *PLOS Medicine.* https://journals.plos.org/plosmedicine/article?id=10.1371/journal.pmed.0010062.
9. Kluge, M., et al. (2007). Ghrelin Administered in the Early Morning Increases Secretion of Cortisol and Growth Hormone Without Affecting Sleep. https://www.sciencedirect.com/science/article/abs/pii/S030645300700011X?via%3Dihub.
10. Lateef, O., & Akintubosun, M. (2020). Sleep and Reproductive Health. https://jcircadianrhythms.com/articles/10.5334/jcr.190.
11. Cai, X.-F., et al. (2024). Association of Sleep Disturbances with Diminished Ovarian Reserve in Women Undergoing Infertility Treatment. *Scientific Reports.* https://www.nature.com/articles/s41598-024-78123-w.
12. Yanik, F., et al. (2024). P-457 The Overlooked Side of Sleep Quality; Can Self-Reported Sleep Quality Have an Impact on the Quality of Oocytes and Embryos in Women Undergoing IVF Treatment? https://academic.oup.com/humrep/article/39/Supplement_1/deae108.805/7703799.
13. Ding, Y., et al. (2024). Relationship Between Sleep Abnormalities and Hypothyroidism: Results from the National Health and Nutrition Examination Survey 2007–2012. https://bmcpublichealth.biomedcentral.com/articles/10.1186/s12889-024-20630-6.
14. Robbins, R., et al. (2020). Four-Year Trends in Sleep Duration and Quality: A Longitudinal Study Using Data from a Commercially Available Sleep Tracker. *Journal of Medical Internet Research.* https://www.jmir.org/2020/2/e14735.

15. Kocevska, D., et al. (2020). Sleep Characteristics Across the Lifespan in 1.1 million People from the Netherlands, United Kingdom and United States: A Systematic Review and Meta-Analysis. *Nature Human Behaviour.* https://www.nature.com/articles/s41562-020-00965-x.
16. Muzni, K., et al. (2020). Self-Reported Sleep Quality Is More Closely Associated with Mental and Physical Health Than Chronotype and Sleep Duration in Young Adults: A Multi-Instrument Analysis. *Journal of Sleep Research.* https://onlinelibrary.wiley.com/doi/10.1111/jsr.13152.
17. Pérez-Medina-Carballo, R., et al. (2023). The Circadian Variation of Sleep and Alertness of Postmenopausal Women. *Sleep.* https://academic.oup.com/sleep/article/46/2/zsac272/6845461.
18. Leng, R., et al. (2025). Influence of Sedentary Behavior on Sleep Quality in Postmenopausal Women in High-Altitude Regions of China: A Cross-Sectional Study. https://www.frontiersin.org/journals/neurology/articles/10.3389/fneur.2024.1476010/full.
19. Soltani, M., et al. (2012). Sleepless Nights: The Effect of Socioeconomic Status, Physical Activity, and Lifestyle Factors on Sleep Quality in a Large Cohort of Australian Women. *Archives of Women's Mental Health.* https://link.springer.com/article/10.1007/s00737-012-0281-3.
20. Zuraikat, F. M., et al. (2020). Measures of Poor Sleep Quality Are Associated With Higher Energy Intake and Poor Diet Quality in a Diverse Sample of Women from the Go Red for Women Strategically Focused Research Network. *Journal of the American Heart Association.* https://www.ahajournals.org/doi/10.1161/JAHA.119.014587.
21. Aygör, H., & Süzer, Ö. (2023). Sleep Quality and Associated Factors in Women. https://dergipark.org.tr/en/pub/bshealthscience/issue/76590/1232307.

22. Wu, X., et al. (2015). Low Physical Activity and High Screen Time Can Increase the Risks of Mental Health Problems and Poor Sleep Quality among Chinese College Students. https://journals.plos.org/plosone/article?id=10.1371/journal.pone.0119607.
23. Sejbuk, M., et al. (2022). Sleep Quality: A Narrative Review on Nutrition, Stimulants, and Physical Activity as Important Factors. *Nutrients*. https://www.mdpi.com/2072-6643/14/9/1912.
24. Agarwal, S. K. (2021). Lifestyles and Their Influence on Sleep Disorders. https://journalindj.com/index.php/INDJ/article/view/311.
25. Sun, T., et al. (2021). Sleep and Circadian Rhythm Disturbances in Intensive Care Unit (ICU)-Acquired Delirium: A Case–Control Study. *The Journal of International Medical Research*, 49. https://doi.org/10.1177/0300060521990502.
26. Leng, R., et al. (2025). Influence of Sedentary Behavior on Sleep Quality in Postmenopausal Women in High-Altitude Regions of China: A Cross-Sectional Study. https://www.frontiersin.org/journals/neurology/articles/10.3389/fneur.2024.1476010/full.
27. Bruni, O., et al. (2021). Herbal Remedies and Their Possible Effect on the GABAergic System and Sleep. *Nutrients*, 13. https://doi.org/10.3390/nu13020530.
28. Donelli, D., et al. (2019). Effects of Lavender on Anxiety: A Systematic Review and Meta-Analysis. *Phytomedicine: International Journal of Phytotherapy and Phytopharmacology*, 65, 153099. https://doi.org/10.1016/j.phymed.2019.153099.
29. Kaźmierczyk, I., et al. (2024). Passiflora incarnata as an Adjunctive Treatment for Anxiety and Sleep Disorders. *Quality in Sport*. https://doi.org/10.12775/qs.2024.35.56361.
30. Kazemi, A., et al. (2024). Effects of Chamomile (*Matricaria chamomilla L.*) on Sleep: A Systematic Review and Meta-Analysis of Clinical Trials. *Complementary Therapies in Medicine*, 103071. https://doi.org/10.1016/j.ctim.2024.103071.

31. Bruni, O., et al. (2021). Herbal Remedies and Their Possible Effect on the GABAergic System and Sleep. *Nutrients*, 13. https://doi.org/10.3390/nu13020530.
32. Xue, L., et al. (2020). A Randomized Controlled Pilot Study of the Effectiveness of Magnolia Tea on Alleviating Depression in Postnatal Women. *Food Science & Nutrition*, 8, 1554–1561. https://doi.org/10.1002/fsn3.1442.
33. Mookiah, S., & Vilva, V. (2025). Sleep-Wake Cycles: Revealing the Hormonal Symphony of Melatonin and Circadian Rhythm Disorders—A Comprehensive Review. *International Journal of Pharmaceutical Sciences and Drug Research*. https://doi.org/10.25004/ijpsdr.2025.170113.
34. Tuft, C., et al. (2023). Current Insights into the Risks of Using Melatonin as a Treatment for Sleep Disorders in Older Adults. *Clinical Interventions in Aging*, 18, 49–59. https://doi.org/10.2147/cia.s361519.
35. Cruz-Sanabria, F., et al. (2024). Optimizing the Time and Dose of Melatonin as a Sleep-Promoting Drug: A Systematic Review of Randomized Controlled Trials and Dose−Response Meta-Analysis. *Journal of Pineal Research*, 76. https://doi.org/10.1111/jpi.12985.
36. Boyle, N., Lawton, C., & Dye, L. (2017). The Effects of Magnesium Supplementation on Subjective Anxiety and Stress—A Systematic Review. *Nutrients*, 9. https://doi.org/10.3390/nu9050429.
37. Hausenblas, H., et al. (2024). Magnesium-L-threonate Improves Sleep Quality and Daytime Functioning in Adults with Self-Reported Sleep Problems: A Randomized Controlled Trial. *Sleep Medicine: X*, 8. https://doi.org/10.1016/j.sleepx.2024.10.121.
38. Cotter, J., et al. (2025). Examining the Effect of L-theanine on Sleep: A Systematic Review of Dietary Supplementation Trials. *Nutritional Neuroscience*, 1–15. https://doi.org/10.1080/1028415x.2025.2556925.

39. Soh, J., et al. (2023). The Effect of Glycine Administration on the Characteristics of Physiological Systems in Human Adults: A Systematic Review. *GeroScience*, 46, 219–239. https://doi.org/10.1007/s11357-023-00970-8.
40. Lu, J., & An, Y. (2018). PO-115 Effects of Phosphatidylserine on Mental States in Elite Shooters. *Exercise Biochemistry Review*. https://doi.org/10.14428/ebr.v1i4.9863.
41. "Sacred Rest: Recover Your Life, Renew Your Energy, Restore Your Sanity." S. Dalton-Smith. 2017. https://www.amazon.com/Sacred-Rest-Saundra-Dalton-Smith-audiobook/dp/B077VS85DS/.

Chapter 9

Balance Your Energy Input and Output

When Sarah first came to see me, she was 38 years old—and hadn't had a period in 20 years. After years of being on and off hormonal birth control and several failed in vitro fertilization (IVF) cycles, her body had quietly shut down. She was tired of being told her hormones were "just confused." Her words to me were "I feel like my body doesn't trust me anymore."

Our goal was simple: get her period back and establish several months of regular, healthy hormone production (her body's own estrogen and progesterone) to feed the health of her uterine lining so that it would be receptive and successful at her next IVF transfer.

After identifying that her lack of a period was due to relative energy deficiency in sport (RED-S), I helped her reignite her body's natural rhythms. We did this not through another medication or aggressive protocol, but by giving her body permission to feel safe again through optimal movement, nourishment, and rest that supported rather than depleted her.

Many women with RED-S, like Sarah, live in a state of quiet depletion that's masked by discipline and drive. They may feel anxious, restless, or irritable when resting, as if slowing down means losing progress. Their self-worth can become tethered to productivity ("I crushed my to-do list"), intense forms of movement ("I'm training for a half-marathon and want to set a new PR"), or body control ("Although I'm embarrassed to admit it, because it sounds so vain and frivolous, when I can't fit into my 'skinny jeans,' I feel really upset").

Over time, chronic under-fueling and overtraining disrupt the brain's serotonin and dopamine signaling, amplifying stress, perfectionism, an overwhelming preoccupation with "eating clean" or achieving a particular fitness level or physique, and obsessive, controlling patterns around food and exercise. While this doesn't always express as a full-blown eating disorder or body dysmorphia, the patterns can still be very disruptive—robbing joy from life. This cycle creates a self-reinforcing loop: the more depleted the body becomes, the more the mind clings to control as a coping strategy.

This psychological landscape mirrors the Achiever hormone type. Achievers often thrive on goals, structure, and high performance, but their nervous systems run in a near-constant state of sympathetic activation. (As you might recall from a previous chapter, sympathetic energy is the highly mobilized, aggressive, fight-or-flight rush that you experience when your nervous system detects an imminent threat. It's useful, in small doses, and when the situation truly calls for it. But when your body is in sympathetic overdrive most of the week, it takes a toll on you.)

Achievers tend to push through fatigue, skip meals, and override their body's cues, interpreting rest as a sign of weakness, a setback, or something they "simply do not have time for." In the context of RED-S, this mindset accelerates hormonal suppression; the body perceives scarcity, while the mind insists on more output.

Healing requires retraining both physiology and psychology: learning that recovery, nourishment, and rest are not losses of discipline but, instead, the path to progress and healing.

From Scarcity to Safety

Within just a few months of working together, Sarah's cycle returned. It stayed consistent for six months. Then, to everyone's joy, she conceived naturally—no interventions needed. She didn't need IVF in the end. She simply needed to re-engage her body's own optimal hormone production and thereby restore her hormone power!

Now, more than a year postpartum, her energy is vibrant, her period is back again and regular, and her labs tell the story of a body that finally feels nourished and safe.

Never underestimate your body's ability to heal when it's given enough energy and the right nutrients. But for your body to heal, it needs to feel safe enough to do so. Restoration doesn't happen when your nervous system feels as though it is under constant threat.

Your Body Longs to Feel Safe: The Connection Between Energy Sufficiency and Hormones

For women, exercise and nutrition aren't just about fitness or aesthetics; they're about *signaling safety* to the brain. Your hormones are constantly evaluating your environment for an answer to a very particular question: "Is there enough energy available to sustain life?"

When the answer is *no*, your body protects you in the most primal way: by pulling energy away from systems that aren't essential for survival, like reproduction, hair growth, and digestion.

This is what happens in RED-S, a condition initially identified in female athletes that was formerly termed the *Female Athlete Triad* but also seen in everyday women and men who are simply doing too much and eating too little.

How Overtraining and Under-Fueling Disrupt Hormones

In women, cortisol, thyroid, insulin, and sex hormones all depend on adequate energy availability. When that balance is off, every system feels the ripple.

- **Cortisol** rises to help liberate stored energy, but chronic elevation leads to fatigue, anxiety, and sleep disruption.
- **Thyroid hormones** slow down metabolism, making it sluggish and lowering body temperature.
- **Estrogen and progesterone** drop, halting ovulation and leading to mood changes, anxiety, or hot-flash-like symptoms even in younger women.
- **Insulin sensitivity** declines, contributing to blood sugar swings and midsection weight gain despite "healthy eating."

Again, these imbalances don't just happen to athletes who train intensely for competitive sports. Any woman who is exerting tons of energy without adequately fueling herself can experience these issues.

Picture a woman who skips breakfast (or eats only a slice of toast with no protein) while rushing to work, speed-walks 15 blocks to her subway stop, stands on her feet for hours each day, and does an evening spin class—all with a nutritional deficit. She may not be an elite athlete, but she is a high performer who is placing tremendous demands on her body without matching them with the right fuel. If she experiences late-night cravings, stubborn weight gain, fatigue, or irritability, it's because she is energetically depleted and hormonally out of whack. Not because she lacks willpower or emotional self-control.

Insufficient Energy = Lack of Safety

You don't have to be training for a marathon or doing CrossFit five days a week to experience RED-S. You just have to be living in a modern world where the body perceives a high level of physiologic stress: overworked, underfed, overstimulated, and under-rested.

For many women, even *four days* of inadequate caloric intake can disrupt their thyroid hormones, lower their luteinizing hormone (LH) pulses, and start to shut down ovulation. Over time, this can lead to functional hypothalamic amenorrhea (FHA), which is the loss of a period due to chronic under-fueling or stress.

This is your body's way of saying: "I don't feel safe enough to reproduce."

The prevention and treatment of this condition are critical not only for fertility but for the long-term health of all women. Hormones like estrogen, progesterone, and testosterone are vital far beyond reproduction. They influence bone density, brain function, cardiovascular health, metabolism, and the integrity of nearly every tissue in the body.

The Other Side of the Spectrum: When Hormones Are Overstimulated

While RED-S represents hormonal suppression due to too little fuel, polyendocrine metabolic ovarian syndrome (PMOS) often represents hormonal dysregulation due to too much stimulation, particularly from insulin and inflammation. It's a reminder that both scarcity and excess can throw our endocrine systems off balance.

PMOS is a hormonal disorder that often causes irregular or missed periods, excess androgen production, and ovaries that develop small, fluid-filled cysts. If you're a woman with PMOS, the wrong combination of diet and movement can amplify the problem. Diets high in saturated fats, refined carbohydrates, and processed foods increase insulin resistance, driving even higher androgen levels and worsening symptoms like acne, irregular cycles, and unwanted hair growth. Sedentary habits compound this, creating a cycle of inflammation, insulin dysregulation, and hormonal chaos.

The research is clear.

In PMOS:

- High saturated fat diets are linked to more severe PMOS symptoms and greater metabolic risk.
- Anti-inflammatory and Mediterranean-style diets rich in fiber, omega-3s, and phytonutrients improve insulin sensitivity, regulate menstrual cycles, and reduce androgen excess.
- Regular exercise, both aerobic and resistance-based, helps restore ovulation, improve mood, and decrease inflammation markers.
- Even modest, consistent movement (walking daily or strength training two to three times per week) can dramatically improve symptoms and reduce long-term metabolic risk.

Just as RED-S teaches us that too little energy can silence the ovaries, PMOS shows us that too much unregulated energy—in the form of glucose and insulin—can overstimulate them. The key is balance: the right nourishment, the right kind of movement, and a lifestyle that supports rhythmic energy use rather than extremes of depletion or overload.

What Midlife Women Need When It Comes to Movement and Food

As women enter their 40s and 50s, hormone fluctuations create a new set of challenges: less estrogen and progesterone, greater cortisol sensitivity, and a natural decline in muscle and bone density. Especially during this stage of a woman's life, the wrong training or nutrition approach can accelerate decline rather than protect vitality.

Dr. Stacy Sims, a renowned exercise physiologist and nutrition scientist specializing in women's health, highlights that women in midlife must train "for the hormones they have, not the ones they used to." Declining estrogen reduces anabolic signaling and recovery capacity, meaning the body becomes less responsive to long-duration cardio or calorie restriction. Instead, midlife women need:

- **Heavy resistance training** (to preserve muscle, bone, and metabolic rate)
- **High-intensity interval bursts** (to maintain cardiovascular health and growth hormone signaling)
- **More protein** (1.8–2.2 g/kg/day, spaced throughout the day to counter anabolic resistance)
- **Sufficient carbohydrates** to stabilize cortisol and prevent nighttime wakefulness
- **Reduced reliance on endurance cardio**, which can elevate stress hormones when estrogen is low

Perimenopausal and menopausal women who under-fuel or overtrain can mimic RED-S physiology, losing muscle, sleep quality, libido, and bone density, even if they're eating "clean." The goal here is to **train smarter, not harder**, with nutrition and exercise that rebuild strength, mitochondrial capacity, and metabolic resilience. The point is that while moving your body is an excellent choice, it's important to consider *how* you're moving and choose options that lead to hormonal balance rather than dysfunction. The workout routine that brings you joy and vitality in your 40s or 50s may look different than it did in your 20s or 30s.

Endocrine Patterns, Challenges, Input/Output Focus

State	Primary Hormonal Pattern	Common Challenge	Movement Focus	Nourishment Focus
RED-S/ FHA	Low estrogen, progesterone, thyroid	Energy scarcity, high cortisol	Restorative + gentle strength	Increase calories, carbs, and minerals
PMOS	High insulin and androgens	Energy overload, poor sensitivity	Resistance + aerobic balance	Anti-inflammatory, low-dietary fats, balanced macros
Perimen-opause/ DOR	Declining estrogen and progesterone	Anabolic resistance, poor recovery	Heavy lifting + HIIT + mobility	Higher protein, steady carbs, support cortisol balance

Whether you're in your 20s optimizing your cycles, your 30s managing stress and fertility, or your 40s and beyond navigating hormonal transition, the principle remains the same: fuel your body thoughtfully so that you're getting just enough food (not too much, not too little), move with intention, and match your energy input to your output.

Muscle: The Endocrine Organ of Longevity

Building and maintaining muscle is one of the most powerful hormone-protective actions you can take. Muscle tissue acts like an endocrine organ, releasing myokines that improve insulin sensitivity, brain function, and inflammation regulation.

Women with greater lean muscle mass have:

- More balanced estrogen metabolism
- Better blood sugar control
- Lower rates of osteoporosis and cognitive decline
- Higher metabolic flexibility and energy

In your 20s, 30s, and 40s, resistance training isn't optional; it's hormonal insurance for your 50s and beyond. Put bluntly, if you want to enjoy flourishing health during the second half of your life, start doing strength training now. This can look like lifting weights at the gym (choose weights that are heavy enough to be challenging but that you can still lift safely, without compromising your form), lifting heavy household items (big jugs of water, canned food, loaded backpack) if you don't have weights available, or doing bodyweight exercises that don't require equipment (push-ups, squats, lunges, and planks).

No gym membership? No problem. Go online and search for "strength training workout, no gym, no equipment," and you'll find thousands of options for at-home workouts, including creative workouts that involve gently cradling your baby or toddler, or even a puppy, and letting them be your "weight" while you do lunges or squats. Highly entertaining for everyone involved! Plus, if there are kids in the room, you're setting a positive example and showing them that movement is an ordinary, regular part of everyday life. They'll grow up with this imprinted in their minds.

The Hypothalamus: Your Hormone CEO

Building muscle matters. Eating enough matters. Resting matters. But the structure coordinating all of it is your hypothalamus.

Think of the hypothalamus as the CEO of your hormonal system. It monitors incoming energy, outgoing energy, stress load, sleep, temperature, and nutrient availability. Its core question is simple:

Is there enough safety and fuel to sustain life?

When energy intake does not match output—whether from overtraining, chronic stress, fasting, illness, or emotional strain—the hypothalamus senses scarcity. In response, it downshifts reproduction and thyroid signaling to conserve resources.

This is the physiology behind:

- RED-S
- FHA
- Stress-driven thyroid suppression
- Low libido and disrupted sleep

In contrast, when insulin and inflammatory signals are chronically elevated—as in PMOS—the hypothalamus receives a different message: overload rather than scarcity. The result is hormonal dysregulation rather than suppression.

During perimenopause and menopause, the CEO is not in crisis—but in transition. Estrogen and progesterone decline. Muscle, recovery capacity, and metabolic flexibility require new strategy. The message remains the same: stability restores balance.

When the hypothalamus feels safe—adequately fueled, sufficiently rested, not chronically threatened—it orchestrates hormone rhythm with remarkable precision.

"Women Are Not Small Men": What Dr. Stacy Sims' Research Teaches

Dr. Stacy Sims' groundbreaking research on the differences between male and female athletes (Sims has published more than 100 peer-reviewed papers and several books) flipped the script on what women actually need from movement and nutrition. Her message is simple: women are not small men. When it comes to exercise and nourishment, women's needs differ from men's in several significant ways.

Our fluctuating hormones change how we metabolize food, recover from training, and respond to stress. Yet most exercise and nutrition models were built on male physiology: steady hormone levels, predictable energy output, and different stress thresholds. Prior to her research, the dominant thinking was that women should eat just like men do (except a little bit less) and should exercise just like men do (except perhaps lift smaller weights). What Sims found is that this thinking is overly simplistic and doesn't account for what women's bodies truly need.

According to Sims' data, women thrive on:

- **Fueling before, during, and after workouts.** Waiting until after training to eat prolongs cortisol elevation and suppresses thyroid and reproductive hormones.
- **Front-loading calories earlier in the day.** Morning and midday meals better support circadian rhythm and blood sugar stability.
- **Regular protein intake.** 20–30 g within 30–60 minutes post-workout supports muscle repair and hormone synthesis.
- **Varied training intensity.** Heavy resistance and sprint work preserve lean muscle, bone density, and metabolic health as estrogen fluctuates.

In short: *eat enough, lift heavy, and rest deeply.*

Cycle-Syncing Versus Cycle-Awareness

You may have heard of cycle-syncing—the practice of aligning food, workouts, and productivity with the phases of your menstrual cycle. The idea is intuitive. Hormones fluctuate across the month. Energy, recovery capacity, and insulin sensitivity shift. Why not work with that rhythm instead of against it?

Does research confirm that cycle syncing leads to improved athletic performance or better overall health? Not really. The science behind *strict* cycle syncing is still limited and mixed.[1] Factors like sleep, stress, and adequate fueling make a much bigger impact on performance and well-being than what phase of your menstrual cycle you are currently in.

Cycle-syncing can empower awareness, but when taken to the extreme, it can also become another form of control. A new set of strict "rules" and "shoulds" that disconnect us from our own signals, and that overcomplicates our lives. Instead, I encourage what I call **cycle-awareness**, using your physiology as feedback, not as a fixed prescription.

Cycle-awareness means tracking your cycle and paying attention to how your body responds to different types of movement, foods, and rest throughout the month. You might notice that high-intensity training feels best in your follicular phase when estrogen is climbing and energy is high, while gentler strength or restorative yoga feels better in the luteal phase when progesterone peaks. You might also notice how your sleep, cravings, or digestion shift across those same weeks. Notice what you feel, and plan your month accordingly, but without being overly rigid. Awareness gives you agency. But always leave room for spontaneity.

You might:

- Increase carbohydrates slightly in the luteal phase if hunger rises
- Schedule more restorative movement during heavier bleeding
- Push performance goals when energy genuinely feels strong
- Eat more iron-rich and iron-containing foods during menses
- Allow more flexibility in your routine and diet midcycle near ovulation

Nourishment as Medicine

Hormones need raw materials, key macronutrients, and micronutrients, and the best ones come from your plate. Restrictive diets, chronic fasting (more on this in a moment), or low-carb plans can deplete the very nutrients needed to make hormones and neurotransmitters.

Macronutrients: The Foundation

Macronutrients are the three primary nutrients your body needs to stay alive and carry on with daily functions: protein, fat, and carbs.

- **Protein:** Provides amino acids, the building blocks for hormones, neurotransmitters, and enzymes. Adequate protein (20–30 g per meal) supports ovulation, thyroid function, lean muscle, and metabolic balance.

  Best sources: eggs, red meat, poultry, fish, lentils, Greek yogurt, tofu, tempeh.
- **Healthy Fats:** Supply cholesterol and essential fatty acids—the scaffolding for estrogen, progesterone, testosterone, and cortisol. Fats also stabilize inflammation and support cell membrane integrity.

  Best sources: olive oil, avocado, nuts, seeds, chia, flax, wild-caught salmon, sardines.
- **Complex Carbohydrates:** Provide steady glucose, the brain's preferred fuel and the hypothalamus's safety signal. Fiber-rich carbs also feed the gut microbiome, which plays a key role in estrogen metabolism and detoxification.

  Best sources: oats, quinoa, lentils, sweet potatoes, berries, apples, and other fruits.

Micronutrients: The Fine-Tuners

Unlike macronutrients, which are needed in large quantities, micronutrients are vitamins that your body needs in small amounts for energy and hormone production.

- **Vitamin A:** Supports ovarian function, cervical mucus production, and gene expression in reproductive tissues.
- **Vitamin D:** Essential for progesterone synthesis, immune regulation, and bone health.
- **Vitamin E:** Protects ovarian follicles and aids progesterone balance.

- **B Vitamins (B1, B2, B3, B5, B6, B7, B9/folate, B12):** Vital cofactors for energy metabolism, neurotransmitter balance, and hormone detoxification.
  - *B6* supports progesterone production and PMS relief.
  - *Folate (B9)* and *B12* aid fertility, methylation, and cell repair.
- **Vitamin C:** Supports adrenal function, collagen synthesis, and iron absorption.
- **Omega-3 Fatty Acids (EPA and DHA):** Reduce inflammation, improve hormone receptor sensitivity, and support brain and mood health.

Minerals: The Messengers and Activators

Like micronutrients, your body needs minerals—in small amounts—to function optimally.

- **Iron and Ferritin:** Support oxygen transport, ovulation, and energy production.
- **Magnesium:** Calms the nervous system, regulates cortisol, and promotes restorative sleep.
- **Zinc:** Key for ovulation, thyroid function, immune strength, and progesterone production.
- **Selenium:** Required for thyroid hormone activation and antioxidant defense in ovarian tissue.
- **Iodine:** Critical for thyroid hormone synthesis and breast health.
- **Copper and Manganese:** Support collagen formation, iron metabolism, and antioxidant enzyme activity.
- **Calcium:** Essential for nerve signaling, muscle contraction, and bone metabolism.

In short, hormones need both *fuel* (macronutrients) and *cofactors* (micronutrients and minerals) to function optimally, not restriction. Chronic fasting, ultra-low-fat diets, or prolonged low-carb plans may look "clean" on paper but often lead to hormonal depletion over time. In addition, it's possible to eat plenty of macronutrients (protein, fat, carbs) and still be taking in adequate energy yet still be missing the micronutrients and minerals your body needs. This can happen when you're eating too much processed food—empty food that delivers calories, but not nutrients. As a result, you are full (perhaps even overly full) but not truly nourished.

A simple mantra: *You cannot heal hormones in a calorie deficit or in nutrient scarcity.*

Intermittent Fasting and Women's Hormones

Intermittent fasting has become popular in recent years, largely due to social media influencers who report that it acts like a reset button for the body, leading to shedding weight quickly, clearing brain fog, reversing the signs of aging, and more. Numerous intermittent fasting approaches have sprung onto the Internet in recent years, with one of the most prevalent being the 16/8 method: fasting for 16 hours per day and eating only during an 8-hour window, such as 10 a.m. to 6 p.m. Other approaches include the 5/2 approach: eating normally for five days of the week and then severely restricting calories on the other two days. Some tout the benefits of alternate-day fasting: fasting for 24 hours, then eating normally for the next 24, and repeating.

Are these methods safe and effective? What does research tell us? Most research on intermittent fasting (IF) and time-restricted eating (TRE) has been done in men or postmenopausal women, so data on cycling women is limited. The evidence suggests fasting can offer some metabolic benefits, but it also carries hormonal risks for women in their reproductive years.

Potential Benefits

Shorter fasting windows (about 10–12 hours) may improve insulin sensitivity, reduce inflammation, and support digestion, particularly when eating patterns align with circadian rhythms (for example, finishing dinner earlier in the evening).[2]

Potential Drawbacks

Longer fasts (beyond 13–14 hours) can raise cortisol, suppress reproductive hormones (GnRH, LH, FSH), and lower thyroid function (T3). This can disrupt ovulation, increase anxiety or sleep issues, and slow metabolism.[3] In women who already have low energy intake or train intensely, fasting may amplify stress and hormonal suppression rather than promote balance.

Dr. Sims summarizes it best: "Women are not small men. Our hormones respond differently to fasting." She emphasizes circadian alignment and consistent fueling over calorie restriction. For most premenopausal women, extended fasting offers few advantages and often backfires. Perimenopausal and postmenopausal women may tolerate slightly longer windows (13–15 hours) if total calories and protein remain adequate, but fasting should never coincide with workouts.

Sims' simple formula: aim for about a 12-hour overnight fast (for example, 7 p.m. to 7 a.m.), break your fast within an hour of waking, and fuel before training. Front-load calories earlier in the day, especially protein, to support cortisol balance, thyroid function, and metabolic health.

When it comes to nourishing yourself effectively, remember these key points:

- **Optimal fasting for most women = 12 hours overnight, not chronic restriction.**
- **Energy availability is non-negotiable.** Fasting is counterproductive if total calorie or protein intake drops too low.
- **Fuel before workouts, especially strength and interval training.** Exercising fasted increases cortisol and blunts recovery.
- **Earlier eating windows (e.g., 7 a.m.–7 p.m.)** better support circadian rhythm, thyroid function, and sleep quality.

- **More fasting isn't better.** Hormonal health depends on consistency, nourishment, and recovery, not deprivation.
- **Caffeine isn't food.** That coffee or tea may give you a temporary jolt or fill up your stomach with liquid, causing you to temporarily feel a sense of satiety, but this is not a meal. Caffeine is a stimulant, not a nutrient. (To the woman who is reading this right now, sipping on her third nonfat milk latte of the day, with a grumbling stomach, this message is for you.)

Hypothalamic Hormone Helpers: Meet the Nootropics

Nourishing yourself means giving yourself adequate fuel (macronutrients, micronutrients, and minerals) to match your energy output (exercise, movement, daily activities). To give your body additional support, one of my favorite categories of hormone helpers are the *nootropics*.

Nootropics are substances that can enhance cognitive functions such as memory, focus, and learning as well as support the CEO of your body: the hypothalamus and pituitary hormone brain centers. Among natural nootropics, several botanicals, vitamins, and amino acids are recognized for their brain-hormone benefits for women. I recommend the following.

Adaptogenic Nootropics

Support the HPA axis and balance the stress–hormone feedback loop to enhance energy, focus, and resilience.

Compound	How It Supports Women's Hormonal Health
Ashwagandha (Withania somnifera)[4]	Calms cortisol, improves sleep, and restores thyroid and reproductive hormone balance
Rhodiola rosea[5]	Enhances mental stamina and reduces fatigue by modulating stress hormones and neurotransmitters

(continued)

(continued)

Compound	How It Supports Women's Hormonal Health
Panax ginseng[6]	Supports energy, libido, and cognitive clarity through gentle estrogen receptor modulation
Holy Basil (Tulsi)[7]	Balances cortisol and blood sugar while easing anxiety and PMS-related mood changes
Schisandra chinensis[8]	Improves endurance, mental clarity, and liver detoxification to enhance estrogen metabolism
Bacopa monnieri[9]	Boosts memory, learning, and focus while reducing oxidative stress in the brain
Vitex (Chaste Tree Berry)[10]	Regulates prolactin and luteal phase progesterone, supporting mood and cycle regularity
Saffron (Crocus sativus)[11]	Elevates mood and relieves PMS or perimenopausal irritability by balancing serotonin and dopamine
L-Theanine[8]	Promotes calm focus and reduces anxiety by increasing alpha brain waves and supporting GABA balance

Nutrient-Based Nootropics

Provide the essential cofactors and building blocks for neurotransmitters, myelin, and hormone synthesis.

Compound	How It Supports Women's Hormonal Health
Choline[12]	Fuels acetylcholine production for memory and supports liver detoxification of estrogen
Iron[11]	Enables oxygen delivery to the brain and ovaries; deficiency impairs cognition and ovulation

Compound	How It Supports Women's Hormonal Health
B-Complex Vitamins (B6, B9/Folate, B12)[13]	Regulate neurotransmitter synthesis, methylation, and progesterone support
Magnesium L-Threonate[14]	Improves brain plasticity, sleep, and stress resilience by calming the HPA axis
Omega-3 Fatty Acids (EPA/DHA)[15]	Reduce inflammation, stabilize mood, and improve hormone receptor sensitivity

Mitochondrial Nootropics

Enhance cellular energy and protect the brain and ovaries from oxidative stress and age-related decline.

Compound	How It Supports Women's Hormonal Health
Creatine[16]	Improves energy, mood, and cognitive performance, particularly in low-estrogen states
Acetyl-L-Carnitine (ALCAR)[17]	Boosts mitochondrial function, mental clarity, and mood regulation during hormonal transitions
Phosphatidylserine[18]	Supports cortisol regulation and memory, helping buffer stress-induced hormonal imbalances
CoQ10 (Ubiquinone/ Ubiquinol)[19]	Enhances mitochondrial energy, fertility, and ovarian reserve while protecting against oxidative stress

Do Lab Testing to Gather More Info

If you suspect RED-S, PMOS, irregular cycles, poor recovery, mood swings, fatigue, or "wired-but-tired" energy, testing provides clarity.

We are not just looking for disease. We are looking for early imbalance.

Which Tests to Do

Collaborating with your provider or healthcare team, check the following labs:

Sex Hormones

Estradiol, progesterone, testosterone (free and total), FSH, LH, SHBG.

Cycle timing matters when applicable.

Thyroid Panel

TSH, Free T3, Free T4 ± antibodies.

Low free T3 or elevated reverse T3 can reflect energy insufficiency or stress suppression.

Cortisol + DHEA-S

A 4-point cortisol panel evaluates rhythm.

Flattened curves or elevated evening cortisol suggest under-recovery or stress overload.

Metabolic Markers

Fasting glucose, HbA1c, fasting insulin.

Insulin dysregulation can amplify PMOS or mimic energy instability.

Iron + Ferritin

Ferritin below ~50 ng/mL can impair thyroid function, ovulation, and energy.

Key Nutrients

Vitamin D, RBC magnesium, B12, zinc.

Micronutrient depletion often accompanies chronic stress or restrictive intake.

Omega-3 Index

Reflects inflammatory balance and hormone receptor sensitivity.

Gut Testing (if indicated)

Consider if digestive symptoms, estrogen metabolism issues, or chronic inflammation are present.

What We're Looking For

- Low progesterone
- Suppressed FSH + LH pulses
- Low estrogen
- Low free T3
- Elevated evening cortisol
- High fasting insulin
- Low ferritin or micronutrient depletion

Re-test after three to four months of consistent nourishment and appropriate training.

Specific Recommendations for the Caretaker, Achiever, and Survivor

Regardless of your Hormone Type, extreme behaviors signal danger to your body. If you are starving your body or over-feeding her, never moving or exercising excessively, these extremes knock your hormones out of whack.

Whether you are a Caretaker, Achiever, or Survivor, the goal is the same: balance the energy you're burning up (through exercise, movement as you go about your day, and bodily functions) with the fuel you're taking in (macronutrients, micronutrients, and minerals). Striking the right balance of output and input signals safety to your body. From this state of safety, your body can bring hormones back to optimal levels, heal, and flourish.

While the end goal is the same, the path to getting there may look different depending on your Hormone Type. The following are my customized recommendations for each type.

The Caretaker

Your Pattern: Caretakers often under-fuel and under-recover because everyone else comes first.

Your Three Highest-Leverage Moves

1. **Eat every three to four hours.**
   Prioritize protein and complex carbohydrates to stabilize cortisol and blood sugar.
2. **Replace intensity with strength.**
   Gentle resistance training and steady walking support muscle without overstimulation.
3. **Affirmation:**
   "When I nourish myself, I strengthen everyone I care for."

The Achiever

Your Pattern: Achievers are most vulnerable to RED-S patterns—overtraining, fasting, caffeine reliance, and pushing through fatigue.

Your Three Highest-Leverage Moves

1. **Cap fasting at 12 hours overnight.**
   Fuel within 60 minutes of waking and before workouts.
2. **Reduce high-intensity frequency.**
   Prioritize heavy lifting with full recovery days over chronic HIIT.
3. **Affirmation:**
   "Steady fuel gives me sustainable power. I am also safe to rest."

The Survivor

Your Pattern: Survivors often oscillate between depletion and stagnation due to chronic stress imprinting.

Your Three Highest-Leverage Moves

1. **Start small and build gradually.**
   Consistent moderate movement signals safety more than extreme bursts.
2. **Increase nutrient density.**
   Protein, omega-3s, iron, magnesium, and B vitamins support stress resilience.
3. **Affirmation:**
   "I am safe to grow stronger at my own pace."

Moderation, Not Perfection

Your body isn't asking for perfection. It only wants you to eat when you're hungry. Rest when you're tired. Move because it feels good, not because you have to "earn" your food or your worth.

When you honor your body's need for energy, rhythm, and safety, your hormones respond with vitality, stability, and ease.

Remember that your body is continually asking, "Am I safe right now? Safe enough to relax? To digest? Ovulate? Reproduce? Repair?" Your job is to reassure your body, "Yes, you are safe." The way that you deliver this message of safety to your body is through steady, reliable nourishment—not starving her, not over-feeding her, not placing unreasonable physical demands on her, and not being sedentary. Instead, ensure that she is well-nourished through appropriate amounts of movement and food—not too much, not too little, just right. The more you do this, the safer your body will feel, and the more you will restore a relationship of trust.

Key Takeaways

- *Sufficient energy = safety.* Your body interprets nourishment as safety. When you move and eat in appropriate amounts—not too little, not too much—you signal to your hormones that it's safe to function optimally.
- *Women are not small men.* Excessive fasting, restrictive eating, and overtraining impact women and men differently. For women, a moderate approach—such as fasting from 7 p.m. to 7 a.m., but not longer than that—best supports hormones and metabolic health.
- *RED-S can result from under-fueling your body, while PMOS can stem from over-fueling.* In both cases, your body interprets the mismatch between energy input and output as "danger." In response, the body shuts down non-essential activities, such as reproduction.
- *Muscle is medicine.* Strength training is one of the most powerful ways to protect hormonal health across your lifespan. Building muscle in your 20s, 30s, and 40s sets you up for greater health in your 50s and beyond, and a smoother transition through menopause.
- *Nourishment isn't about perfection—it's about moderation and equilibrium.* It's not about eating "clean" all the time or adhering to the "perfect" workout routine. It's about creating balance—replenishing yourself with macronutrients, micronutrients, minerals, and movement that makes you feel powerful. And, making sure you are taking in as much fuel as you burn.

Notes

1. Hackney, A., Hansen, M., & Melin, A. (2025). Menstrual Cycle Effects on Sports Performance and Adaptations to Training: A Historical Perspective. *Scandinavian Journal of Medicine & Science in Sports*, 35. https://doi.org/10.1111/sms.70107.
2. Ciastek, B., Kapłon, K., & Domaszewski, P. (2025). A Comprehensive Perspective on the Biological Effects of Intermittent Fasting and Periodic Short-Term Fasting: A Promising Strategy for Optimizing Metabolic Health. *Nutrients*, 17. https://doi.org/10.3390/nu17132061.
3. Kim, B., et al. (2021). Effects of Intermittent Fasting on the Circulating Levels and Circadian Rhythms of Hormones. *Endocrinology and Metabolism*, 36, 745–756. https://doi.org/10.3803/enm.2021.405.
4. Haddad, S., & Houssaini, M. (2025). Effects of Ashwagandha Supplements on Cortisol, Stress, and Anxiety Levels in Adults: A Systematic Review and Meta-Analysis. *BJPsych Open*, 11, S39–S39. https://doi.org/10.1192/bjo.2025.10136.
5. Stojcheva, E., & Quintela, J. (2022). The Effectiveness of *Rhodiola rosea* L. Preparations in Alleviating Various Aspects of Life-Stress Symptoms and Stress-Induced Conditions—Encouraging Clinical Evidence. *Molecules*, 27. https://doi.org/10.3390/molecules27123902.
6. Jahan, F., et al. (2025). Unlocking Nature's Potential: The Power of Adaptogens in Enhancing Modern Health and Wellness. *Journal of Agriculture and Food Research*. https://doi.org/10.1016/j.jafr.2025.102501.
7. Lopresti, A., et al. (2021). Modulation of the Hypothalamic–Pituitary–Adrenal (HPA) Axis by Plants and Phytonutrients: A Systematic Review of Human Trials. *Nutritional Neuroscience*, 25, 1704–1730. https://doi.org/10.1080/1028415x.2021.1892253.
8. Chan, S. (2012). Panax Ginseng Rhodiola Rosea and Schisandra Chinensis. *International Journal of Food Sciences and Nutrition*, 63, 75–81. https://doi.org/10.3109/09637486.2011.627840.

9. Tóth-Mészáros, et al. (2023). The Effect of Adaptogenic Plants on Stress: A Systematic Review and Meta-Analysis. *Journal of Functional Foods*. https://doi.org/10.1016/j.jff.2023.105695.
10. Bharti, K., et al. (2025). Natural Compounds for Mental Wellness: A Focus on Neuroprotective and Adaptogenic Effects. *Journal of Dynamics and Control*. https://doi.org/10.71058/jodac.v9i7012.
11. Tardy, A., et al. (2020). Vitamins and Minerals for Energy, Fatigue and Cognition: A Narrative Review of the Biochemical and Clinical Evidence. *Nutrients*, 12. https://doi.org/10.3390/nu12010228.
12. Kansakar, U., et al. (2023). Choline Supplements: An Update. *Frontiers in Endocrinology*, 14. https://doi.org/10.3389/fendo.2023.1148166.
13. Businaro, R. (2022). Food Supplements to Complement Brain Functioning: The Benefits of a Combination of Magnesium, Folic Acid, Omega-3 Fatty acids and Vitamin E. *F1000Research*.
14. Carvalho, J., et al. (2024). Exploring Cognitive Trails: A Review on the Benefits of Supplementation on Cognition and Mental Performance. *International Journal of Health Science*. https://doi.org/10.22533/at.ed.159432409013.
15. Businaro, R. (2022). Food Supplements to Complement Brain Functioning: The Benefits of a Combination of Magnesium, Folic Acid, Omega-3 Fatty Acids and Vitamin E. *F1000Research*. https://doi.org/10.12688/f1000research.75856.1.
16. Walczak, K., et al. (2024). Effect of Creatine Supplementation on Cognitive Function and Mood. *Journal of Education, Health and Sport*. https://doi.org/10.12775/jehs.2024.73.51712.
17. Pennisi, M., et al. (2020). Acetyl-L-Carnitine in Dementia and Other Cognitive Disorders: A Critical Update. *Nutrients*, 12(5), 1389. https://doi.org/10.3390/nu12051389. PMID: 32408706; PMCID: PMC7284336.

18. Starks, M. A., et al. (2008). The Effects of Phosphatidylserine on Endocrine Response to Moderate Intensity Exercise. *Journal of the International Society of Sports Nutrition*, 5, 11. https://doi.org/10.1186/1550-2783-5-11. PMID: 18662395; PMCID: PMC2503954.
19. Jiang, Y., et al. (2025). Exploring the Protective Effects of Coenzyme Q10 on Female Fertility. *Frontiers in Cell and Developmental Biology*, 13, 1633166. https://doi.org/10.3389/fcell.2025.1633166. PMID: 40950399; PMCID: PMC12425901.

Chapter 10

Support Detoxification and Fight Chronic Inflammation

Miriam, a 39-year-old woman, came to me after four heartbreaking pregnancy losses. All the standard workup through a top reproductive endocrinology clinic had come back normal. Genetics? Normal. Fertility labs? Normal. Imaging? Normal. She was told everything "looked fine" and was referred to me to "think outside the box."

When she sat in my office, she quietly said something that stuck with me:

> "I feel terrible in my house. I don't know how else to explain it."

That sentence changed the entire trajectory of her care.

She described fatigue, as well as rashes, headaches, sneezing, and itchy eyes—symptoms of inflammation that began shortly after moving into her home in Southeast Portland. At first, she waved it off ("It's probably just seasonal allergies. Portland is bursting with flowers and pollen in the spring. . ."), but the symptoms persisted year-round. All the aching and sniffling started after she moved into her new home. That's when the pregnancy losses began, too. She hadn't connected the two events, and none of her healthcare providers had connected the dots either.

Alarm bells went off in my mind. *Environmental toxins. Impaired detoxification. Chronic inflammation.*

By digging deeper and doing lab testing to confirm my hunch, we uncovered elevated inorganic arsenic on her 24-hour urine test. Miriam was slowly being poisoned to death. No wonder she was having difficulty conceiving. Her body was incompatible with life.

The cause? Turns out, her house was in a known exposure zone near a glass factory, a hot zone for arsenic and cadmium exposure due to a factory leak. On top of that, water damage in her home (Portland is one of the rainiest cities in the United States) created mold and mildew, which she inhaled daily, further exacerbating her condition. She moved out, rebuilt her nutrient terrain, supported her liver and gut to promote detoxification, and reduced inflammation. Her next IUI resulted in a full-term pregnancy and healthy delivery.

I'm grateful we were able to turn her negative trajectory around. I only wish it could have happened sooner, sparing her years of poor health and tragic losses that might have been prevented.

You may not be experiencing toxicity to the same degree that Miriam was. Her case was on the more extreme end of the spectrum. However, millions of women are dealing with their own version of detoxification issues and inflammation. I see it in my clinic, week after week, and if there's one universal truth that I know, it is this:

You cannot have stable hormones in an inflamed body with an overburdened detox system.

Fortunately, there are powerful, evidence-backed actions you can take to support your body's natural detoxification systems, while limiting your exposure to toxins as best you can.

It's not about doing everything perfectly. It's about doing a few things consistently. That's what this chapter is all about.

The Truth About Detoxification

When you hear the word *detox*, you might envision a social media influencer describing her 30-day juice cleanse and how fasting and sipping nothing but celery juice, while also doing daily enemas, changed her life. This is *not* what I recommend, nor is it what detoxification means from a medical perspective. The word *detox* has gotten a bad rap due to misinformation being spread online. (While many content creators have good intentions and hope to help and inspire others, it's essential to make sure you're getting healthcare information from qualified sources.)

Detoxification and inflammation are not fringe wellness concepts. They are core physiologic processes that decide how your hormones behave. Estrogen and progesterone especially rely on optimal detoxification, especially for maintaining hormonal balance and reducing disease risk. But cortisol, thyroid, insulin, and many other core hormones also rely on a healthy liver, microbiome, and immune system. When these systems are stressed, hormone stress follows.

Your Body's Built-In Detox Systems

Your body was designed with natural, built-in systems to handle detoxification beautifully. To give you a quick overview. . .

- Your **skin**, the largest organ in your body, provides an external barrier to reduce the amount of toxins that can penetrate your body.
- Your **lungs** provide an air filtration system: mucus inside your lungs traps dust, bacteria, viruses, and other foreign particles. Little hair-like appendages called cilia sweep up these foreign particles so you can cough them up or sneeze them out. Cells called macrophages neutralize any remaining particles that the cilia miss.
- Your **digestive system** compels you to vomit if you accidentally ingest something toxic, purging it from your body before it can harm you too much.
- Your **kidneys** filter waste and toxins from your blood.
- Your **liver** also detoxifies your blood, breaking down harmful substances, so they can eventually be excreted in bile or urine.

Your body has other organs and systems that aid in detoxification, too, but that's a brief glimpse at how the process works. It's a brilliant design. All these systems are working 365 days a year, 24/7, to detoxify your body and keep things humming optimally.

So, detoxification doesn't mean drinking vegetable juice for a week to "cleanse" yourself. It means supporting your body's natural detox pathways so they can do their job effectively, while reducing the strain on these systems by reducing the quantity of toxins entering your system.

You may be wondering, "If human bodies are built to detox naturally, why do we need to actively support detox? Shouldn't my body just be able to handle things on its own?"

To answer: Yes, your body already detoxifies. It has exquisite detoxification systems in place, built into your skin, in every breath you take, and beyond. But modern life places a load on those systems that they were never designed to manage, including:

- Increased exposure to endocrine-disrupting chemicals
- Chronic stress and cortisol dysregulation

- Sedentary lifestyles
- Ultra-processed food and alcohol use
- Environmental pollutants
- Microbiome depletion from medications and antibiotics
- Sleep loss
- Excessive workload and screen time
- Chronic low-grade or high-grade inflammation

So yes, your body is designed with systems to naturally detoxify itself. But these systems can handle only so much. At a certain point, they buckle under the strain of modern life and struggle to work effectively.

Imagine a bathtub, a metaphor we will revisit later, that is designed with a drain, but someone keeps dumping mud and sludge into the tub, buckets at a time, faster than the drain can handle. The system is overloaded. This is what happens for many of the women I treat: their body's detox systems are overwhelmed and can't keep up with the demands being placed on them. And this strain can directly translate into hormonal symptoms and hormone disruption: PMS, heavy bleeding, breast tenderness, mood swings, fatigue, stubborn weight gain, migraines, acne, bloating, and the classic estrogen-dominance, or rather, progesterone-deficient pattern I see constantly.

Supporting detoxification is not about "flushing toxins" from your body using extreme measures. It's about giving your liver and gut the resources they need to keep up with the hormonal and environmental demands of modern life.

What Is Inflammation?

Inflammation is your body's alarm system. When it's acute, it protects you. When it becomes chronic, it drives hormonal chaos from low progesterone to insulin resistance, PMS, heavy bleeding, migraines, breast tenderness, anxiety, and stubborn weight gain.

Sometimes, inflammation is visible and obvious, an angry rash, acne, or puffy-looking face. Other times, it's invisible. Think: digestive distress, joint pain, or fatigue.

Acute inflammation is temporary, short-lived, and serves an important purpose. When you scrape your knee on a hike and the surrounding skin becomes red and swells up a bit, this is acute inflammation—a sign that your body's natural healing systems are at work. Chronic inflammation is different. It's when there is too much inflammation, for too long, which signals, "The body's detox systems are overloaded and need support. They can't keep up with the workload."

Lowering inflammation is not about doing everything perfectly. It's about doing a few things consistently.

Top Causes of Chronic Inflammation in Women

Chronic inflammation is not random. It is usually driven by a handful of predictable patterns that show up again and again in my clinic: hormonal, metabolic, autoimmune, and lifestyle factors that keep the body in a low-grade or high-grade inflammatory state. I will go deeper into these drivers in Chapter 11, but you need to see them here, because the strategies in this chapter are the foundation of care in all these cases.

Here are the major causes of chronic inflammation in most women:

PMOS

Insulin resistance and androgen excess create a self-reinforcing inflammatory loop. Inflammation worsens hormone imbalance, which worsens metabolic strain.

Endometriosis

An estrogen-driven, immune-mediated condition characterized by inflammatory cytokine signaling. Pain is only part of the story; systemic inflammation is the terrain.

Body composition and inflammatory adiposity
Visceral fat functions like an inflammatory endocrine organ, producing cytokines that drive insulin resistance and hormone disruption. Body composition matters more than BMI.

Menopause and aging
As estrogen declines, its anti-inflammatory protection declines as well. Metabolic and vascular risk can rise during this transition. We will explore this more as well as discuss risk factors and cases of premature ovarian insufficiency (POI)/early menopause in Chapter 11.

Autoimmune conditions
Chronic immune activation influences thyroid signaling, hormone receptors, and energy production.

Stress and poor sleep
Elevated cortisol and circadian disruption amplify inflammatory mediators, especially in women balancing caregiving and career demands.

Environmental and lifestyle factors
Ultra-processed food, excess sugar and alcohol, sedentary time, pollution, indoor air contaminants, and chronic psychological stress all layer on top of these other drivers. They increase oxidative stress, burden the liver, alter the microbiome, and amplify inflammatory pathways.

Most women have more than one of these factors operating at the same time. That is why you cannot "spot treat" or take a single supplement to treat inflammation. You need strategies that lower inflammatory load, support detoxification, nourish the gut, strengthen the internal terrain, and that are personalized to the individual. Next, we will look at how environmental medicine fits into this picture.

Meet Environmental Medicine: The Missing Piece in Women's Hormone Care

Before I share the best practices to support detox and fight chronic inflammation, it's essential to understand a key (and too often missed) reason why so many women struggle in the first place. And that begins with *environmental medicine.*

Environmental medicine examines how chemicals, pollutants, microbes, and physical hazards in our air, water, food, and homes interact with human physiology. It sits at the intersection of toxicology, genetics, immunology, and microbiome science. And it directly influences hormone function.

In all my years supporting women, environmental factors were rarely part of prior workups—even in cases of recurrent pregnancy loss. Yet endocrine-disrupting chemicals can alter estrogen signaling, mitochondrial function, thyroid activity, and immune regulation.

I have seen this repeatedly.

Another patient in her early 30s came to me with painful PMS and infertility despite "normal" labs. When we assessed her environment, the picture shifted: daily cooking on scratched nonstick pans, fragranced cleaning products, water damage at work, and high-traffic exposure near her home. We focused on improving air and water quality, replacing cookware and synthetic fragrances, increasing cruciferous vegetables and fiber, and supporting glutathione pathways. Within six months, her PMS resolved, and she conceived naturally.

Environmental medicine is not fringe. It is foundational.

We cannot avoid every toxin. In the United States alone, tens of thousands of chemicals are in circulation. The risk is cumulative. But two women with identical exposures may respond differently.

The difference is terrain.

When liver function, gut integrity, antioxidant systems, and mitochondrial resilience are strong, the body can handle far more than we give it credit for.

We can't avoid every toxin, but we can fortify our biology to handle them. This is the empowering message that women need to hear. It puts women back in the center of their health story. And this is where detox physiology comes in.

Next, I'll share how to strengthen your inner terrain so that you can keep your hormones supported, even in a modern world that isn't getting any cleaner.

It's Not Just About Avoiding Toxins

If you can avoid environmental toxicants, great. This helps tremendously. But the truth is, it's not possible to avoid every single pollutant or harmful chemical in the world. We have to do our best to remove and reduce, but that's why it's also essential to focus on other action steps, too—ones that strengthen and fortify your body's natural detox systems.

Here's what the research shows. . .

Cruciferous Vegetables Boost Your Body's Detox Powers[1]

Sulforaphane from broccoli sprouts increases detoxification of airborne pollutants by up to 61% in human studies. Cruciferous vegetables are rich in glucosinolates, which are converted during chewing and digestion into bioactive compounds like isothiocyanates (notably sulforaphane) and indoles. This process enhances the body's ability to detoxify carcinogens and reactive oxygen species, providing cellular protection.

Fiber Reduces Toxin Recirculation[2]

High-fiber diets bind pesticides, heavy metals, and excess estrogens, reducing their absorption and increasing excretion. Dietary fiber helps lower toxin recirculation by reshaping the gut environment, strengthening the intestinal barrier, and promoting elimination.

Fiber feeds beneficial gut bacteria, increasing short-chain fatty acids that reduce the production and absorption of harmful metabolites like indoxyl sulfate and p-cresyl sulfate. Certain fibers can bind toxins and their precursors directly in the gut, increasing fecal excretion.

Some fibers, such as psyllium, also bind bile acids and other compounds, interrupting enterohepatic recirculation and further reducing toxin load.

Omega-3s Buffer Inflammation from Pollutants[3,4]

Omega-3 fatty acids, found in salmon, mackerel, walnuts, chia seeds, and flaxseeds, help quiet inflammation by lowering pro-inflammatory cytokines, inhibiting key inflammatory pathways, and serving as building blocks for specialized pro-resolving mediators that actively turn off inflammation. They also modulate immune cell activity toward a more anti-inflammatory state and reduce oxidative stress.

Research shows that omega-3 intake can lessen the inflammatory and oxidative effects of air pollutants like particulate matter and ozone, and emerging evidence suggests they may also help buffer some immune and thyroid effects of heavy metal exposure.

Polyphenols Enhance Antioxidant Defenses[5,6]

Polyphenols, compounds found in berries, olive oil, green tea extract, rosemary, and pomegranate, strengthen mitochondrial resilience and lower oxidative stress.

Exercise Increases Glutathione and Toxin Clearance[7]

Regular movement boosts lymphatic flow, improves hepatic blood flow, and enhances detoxification. Exercise boosts glutathione, the body's master antioxidant, by activating glutathione-related enzymes, increasing its synthesis and recycling, and enhancing the body's ability to neutralize oxidative stress and support toxin clearance.

A Healthy Microbiome Aids Detox[8,9]

Beneficial gut bacteria help break down chemicals, reduce beta-glucuronidase, and prevent estrogen from recirculating. A healthy gut microbiome plays a major role in detoxification by breaking down chemicals, regulating estrogen metabolism, and protecting the gut barrier.

Fill, Wash, Drain: The Three Phases of Detoxification[10,11,12,13,14]

Now that you understand why detox is essential, let's talk about how it works in your body. From a physiological standpoint, detoxification happens in three phases. I like to describe the process like a bathtub.

- **Phase 1** is the faucet filling the tub.
- **Phase 2** is when the soap goes in, and you wash off the dirt.
- **Phase 3** is when you pull the plug, and the dirty water drains out.

For everything to work smoothly, three things must happen:

1. The water coming in needs to be at a manageable flow.
2. The soap and water need to remove the dirt.
3. The drain needs to be fully open so the dirty water can leave.

If the faucet is turned up too high, the water rises faster than the drain can handle. If there is no soap, the dirt stays stuck to your skin. If the drain is clogged, the water becomes murky and overflows.

Detoxification works the same way. Your liver, gallbladder, bile ducts, gut, kidneys, skin, and lymphatic system are all working together to transform hormones and toxicants, neutralize them, and eliminate them from your body.

When any phase is overwhelmed, under-fueled, or blocked, symptoms show up.

Phase 1: Turning on the Faucet (Liver Activation)

Phase 1 is when your liver enzymes first interact with hormones, medications, and environmental chemicals. They use oxidation, reduction, and hydrolysis reactions to partially break these substances down and make them ready for the next phase.

This step is essential, but it generates a lot of free radicals. When free radicals build up excessively in the body, they can damage cells which leads to premature aging and developing certain diseases. That means Phase 1 needs antioxidant support so that the "water" flowing into the tub does not damage the tissues around it.

Signs That Phase 1 May Be out of Balance

- Strong reactions to caffeine, alcohol, or medications
- Headaches or nausea with certain smells or chemicals
- Feeling worse with aggressive "detoxes"

How to Support Phase 1

Lifestyle:

- Eat color-rich plant foods every day: berries, leafy greens, beets, carrots, peppers
- Reduce or eliminate alcohol for a season or forever
- Choose organic options for high-pesticide produce when possible
- Spend time outside and breathe fresh air
- Decrease exposure to synthetic fragrances and harsh cleaning agents

Nutrients:

- N-Acetyl Cystine (NAC)
- Glutathione
- B vitamins (especially B2, B3, B6, B12, folate)
- Zinc
- Milk thistle and other liver-supportive herbs

Your goal in Phase 1 is not to "speed up detox" at all costs. It is to keep the faucet flowing at a pace your body can handle, with enough antioxidant support to protect your cells.

Phase 2: Adding the Soap (Conjugation)

Phase 2 is where your liver attaches helper molecules to the Phase 1 products. This is called *conjugation*. These attachments make substances more water-soluble, less reactive, and easier to excrete. Think of this like adding soap and scrubbing the skin so the dirt lifts off and goes into the bathwater.

Phase 2 uses several main pathways: glucuronidation, glutathione conjugation, sulfation, methylation, and amino acid conjugation. Each pathway depends on specific nutrients and amino acids.

Signs That Phase 2 May Need Support

- Estrogen dominance symptoms like heavy bleeding, breast tenderness, and PMS
- Sensitivity to chemicals, fragrances, or medications
- Histamine intolerance or flushing reactions

How to Support Phase 2

Lifestyle:

- Eat enough protein to supply amino acids like glycine, taurine, and cysteine.
- Include cruciferous vegetables such as broccoli, Brussels sprouts, kale, cabbage, and broccoli sprouts.
- Add flavonoid-rich foods like berries, citrus, onions, herbs, and green tea.
- Stay well hydrated so conjugated toxins have fluid to move in.

Nutrients:

- Glycine
- Cysteine or NAC
- Alpha-lipoic acid
- B vitamins that support methylation
- Ellagic acid and other polyphenols

When Phase 2 is happening as it should, the "soap" is plentiful and effective. Hormones like estrogen are packaged in a safer, more excretable form instead of recirculating in ways that cause symptoms.

Phase 3: Pulling the Plug (Elimination and Drainage)

Phase 3 is all about getting the dirty water out of the tub. Once hormones and toxicants have been modified and conjugated, they need to be transported out of the liver via bile or blood and then eliminated through stool, urine, and sweat.

If the drain is slow or clogged, everything backs up. The bathtub is full of soapy, dirty water, and your body starts to reabsorb what you were trying to get rid of.

Phase 3 Depends On

- Healthy bile flow from the liver and gallbladder
- Regular, complete bowel movements (avoiding constipation)
- Good kidney function and hydration
- Sweating and lymphatic circulation

Signs That Phase 3 May Be Sluggish

- Constipation or incomplete bowel movements
- Bloating, feeling "backed up" or heavy
- Worsening symptoms with hormone shifts
- Feeling puffy, swollen, or waterlogged

How to Support Phase 3

Lifestyle:

- Eat a high-fiber diet with plenty of vegetables, legumes, seeds, and whole foods.
- Drink enough water throughout the day.
- Move your body daily to support lymph and bowel motility.
- Aim for at least one full, formed bowel movement daily.
- Use practices that increase sweating when appropriate, such as brisk walking or sauna.

Nutrients:

- Calcium D-glucarate to support estrogen elimination
- Ginger and other motility-supporting herbs
- Melatonin to support gut motility and sleep
- NAC to maintain glutathione and bile quality
- Binders (such as certain clays or charcoal) used thoughtfully and under guidance when indicated

When all three phases are supported, the bathtub works the way it should: clean water in, dirt lifted off, dirty water out. Inflammation calms, hormones become more predictable, and symptoms often improve.

Putting It into Practice

Once you understand the three phases of detox, the question becomes, "Now what? What should I do with this information?"

In my clinic, the most effective plans are never about extreme interventions. Instead, we start with a strong foundation, built on the least-invasive options first.

Here are the big steps to put into practice: one, upgrade your lifestyle and diet to strengthen your body's detox systems. Two, support gut health. Three, clean up environmental toxins as much as possible. If those three steps don't yield the results you're hoping for, consider higher-level interventions for an added boost.

1. Upgrade Your Lifestyle and Diet

You cannot out-supplement a lifestyle that constantly pushes your detox and inflammatory systems into overdrive.

Key actions (much of this we have already covered in prior chapters, so consider this a quick review):

- Build meals around protein, fiber, and healthy fats so blood sugar is stable.
- Aim for at least two cups of vegetables at most meals, with one serving of cruciferous vegetables daily.
- Choose a Mediterranean-style diet whenever possible: olive oil, fish, legumes, nuts, seeds, vegetables, fruit, herbs, and spices.
- Hydrate with clean water throughout the day.
- Limit or remove alcohol, especially if you already have hormonal symptoms or liver strain.
- Prioritize 7–9 hours of sleep at night (ideally between 10 p.m. to 6 a.m.) to allow repair and detox processes to do their work.
- Move your body most days of the week, alternating strength training, walking, and gentle movement.

Scan the code to download my **21-Day Clean Eating and Lifestyle Guide**. It's not a fast. Not a juice cleanse. Not a diet. Nothing restrictive or extreme. Just sensible options to support your body's built-in detox pathways.

2. Support Gut Health

The gut is not just a digestion tube. It is a hormone-processing center, a major immune organ, and home to the estrobolome that regulates how estrogen is metabolized. When the gut is inflamed or imbalanced, hormones cannot communicate clearly.

To restore the Gut-Brain-Hormone communication axis:

- **Get a thorough gut assessment when needed**
  This might include:
  - A detailed symptom and diet history
  - Targeted stool testing (infection panel + microbiome + digestive markers)
  - Assessment for SIBO, H. pylori, or pathologic or opportunistic overgrowths
  - Imaging when indicated for structural concerns

- **Restore the microbiome**
  Depending on what we find, this may mean:
  - Removing irritants and triggering foods
  - Treating infections or overgrowths
  - Incorporating probiotics, prebiotics, and occasionally postbiotics
  - Emphasizing fiber and polyphenol-rich foods

- **Establish long-term gut habits**
  - Do not go too long without eating during the day.
  - Avoid eating large meals close to bedtime.
  - Eat in a relaxed, present state as often as possible.
  - Choose local, organic, minimally processed foods when you can.

Clinically, when gut lining integrity and microbial balance are restored, women often report better mood stability, more regular cycles, steadier energy, and more resilience to stress. This is part of the terrain we are building.

3. Clean Up Exposure to Environmental Toxicants

While we cannot avoid every toxin, we can significantly lighten the load.

High-impact areas to start the cleanup:

- Switch to fragrance-free or naturally scented cleaning and personal care products.
- Replace nonstick cookware with stainless steel, cast iron, or ceramic.
- Filter drinking and cooking water with a high-quality filter.
- Store food in glass or stainless steel instead of plastic when possible.
- Reduce pesticide exposure by choosing organic and washing produce well.
- Improve indoor air quality by ventilating, using air filters as needed, and addressing any water damage or mold promptly.

Scan to find the Environmental Toxin Guide, a self-assessment to help you identify your top exposure sources and take the next right step.

Consider Higher-Level Interventions—As Needed

For many women, the three steps I just mentioned create powerful changes. For others, especially those with more complex conditions, we layer in higher-level support, including botanicals and nutrient supplements.

These are a few that I commonly prescribe to support detox and reduce inflammation (always speak with your healthcare provider before adding supplements to your routine):

- Milk thistle, artichoke, dandelion, and burdock to support liver function and bile flow
- Curcumin and Boswellia to calm inflammation
- Green tea extract, rosemary, and resveratrol for antioxidant and detox support
- NAC, glycine, and alpha-lipoic acid to support glutathione and Phase 2 pathways
- Calcium D-glucarate for estrogen clearance
- Magnesium for motility, nervous system regulation, and detox pathways
- High-quality individualized prebiotics, probiotics, and occasionally postbiotics tailored to gut patterns
- Omega-3 fatty acids for inflammatory balance and hormone support

I highly recommend meeting with a clinician trained in endocrine, gastroenterology, and/or environmental medicine, or a naturopathic doctor with these areas of expertise, if you suspect or know you have:

- Significant mold exposure or chronic inflammatory response syndrome
- Histamine intolerance or mast cell activation syndrome (MCAS)
- Chronic, unexplained fatigue with multi-system symptoms
- Heavy metal exposure
- Cholestasis or significant liver disease
- Inflammatory bowel disease or complex gut conditions

These situations often require careful pacing, more advanced testing, and a personalized plan that considers your unique terrain.

Specific Recommendations for the Caretaker, Achiever, and Survivor

Women metabolize toxins differently depending on their physiology and their patterns of living. Three women—a Caretaker, Achiever, and Survivor—could all be exposed to the same sources of stress, and the same environmental toxins, even living in the same house, yet react in different ways. This is why personalizing your plan is key.

The following are my recommendations for each Hormone Type.

The Caretaker

Your Pattern: As a Caretaker, you might care deeply about protecting your loved ones (purchasing natural, organic, BPA- and phthalate-free products for your children, for example), but when it comes to yourself, you skimp on care.

Your Three Highest-Leverage Moves

1. **Support Phase 3 daily.**
   Hydrate consistently, eat fiber-rich meals with cruciferous vegetables, and aim for one complete bowel movement each day to prevent estrogen recirculation.
2. **Stabilize your rhythm.**
   Eat a nourishing breakfast, walk after meals, and choose steady movement over extremes to calm inflammation and support bile flow.
3. **Affirmation:**
   "I can gently support my body in doing what it was designed to do."

The Achiever

Your Pattern: Achievers often overload Phase 1 detox with stress, caffeine, alcohol, and intensity—creating oxidative strain and hormonal imbalance.

Your Three Highest-Leverage Moves

1. **Lower your oxidative load.**
   Reduce alcohol and excess caffeine, increase colorful plant foods, and support antioxidant pathways through rest and recovery.
2. **Choose moderation over extremes.**
   Avoid aggressive detox tactics. Build strength, schedule recovery days, and let your liver work at a sustainable pace.
3. **Affirmation:**
   "My body detoxifies best when I choose balance over extremes."

The Survivor

Your Pattern: Adrenal depletion, blood sugar dysregulation, sluggish digestion, low vitality—out of the three Hormone Types, Survivors tend to struggle with detoxification and inflammation issues the most.

Your Three Highest-Leverage Moves

1. **Rebuild your internal terrain.**
   Eat three steady meals daily with adequate protein and omega-3s to support glutathione production and stabilize blood sugar.
2. **Move gently and consistently.**
   Walking, light strength work, and practices that support sweating and lymph flow strengthen elimination without overwhelming your system.
3. **Affirmation:**
   "I can rebuild my resilience, one steady step at a time."

Consistency, Not Perfection

Supporting detoxification and lowering inflammation is not about doing everything perfectly. It's about doing a few things consistently.

Toxins are everywhere. That's the reality of the world we live in. You can't live in a bubble and avoid every single source of potential toxins (restaurants, car washes, roads, hotels, airports...) nor do you need to. Your body was intelligently designed to handle a great deal of toxicity. But it does have its limits and can only do so much.

Reduce exposure to harmful substances, to a reasonable extent, while fortifying your body's ability to detoxify itself. Small choices, done consistently, allow your body to do exactly what it was designed to do.

Key Takeaways

- Your body was designed to detoxify itself—but modern life (stress, lack of sleep, poor diet, environmental toxins, etc.) can sometimes overwhelm your body with "too much work to do."
- When your body is overwhelmed, inflammation arises, serving as nature's alarm system. "Hey, something needs to change!"
- Chronic inflammation = too much inflammation, for too long. PMS, heavy bleeding, mood swings, fatigue, and a host of other issues arise.
- Supporting detox and fighting inflammation requires reducing toxins as much as you can, while fortifying your body's built-in systems.

- You don't need extreme measures (like a celery juice fast, or hours in a sweat lodge) to detoxify and reduce inflammation. Stick to the basics: move often, hydrate well, load up on fiber-rich foods including veggies, make gut-friendly choices, get enough sleep, and minimize environmental toxins to the extent that you can. Add in targeted botanicals and nutrients as needed, with your healthcare provider's sign-off.
- You don't need a 100% "clean" or "pure" lifestyle to balance your hormones and achieve optimal health. Make positive lifestyle choices most of the time and let your body handle the occasional deviations as it was meant to do.

Notes

1. Esteve, M. (2020). Mechanisms Underlying Biological Effects of Cruciferous Glucosinolate-Derived Isothiocyanates/ Indoles: A Focus on Metabolic Syndrome. *Frontiers in Nutrition*. https://www.frontiersin.org/journals/nutrition/articles/ 10.3389/fnut.2020.00111/full.
2. Xie, L., et al. (2023). A Major Mechanism for Immunomodulation: Dietary Fibres and Acid Metabolites. *Seminars in Immunology*. https://www.sciencedirect.com/science/article/abs/ pii/S1044532323000283?via%3Dihub.
3. Ma, J., et al. (2025). Omega-3 Modify the Adverse Effects of Long-Term Exposure to Ambient Air Pollution on the Incidence of Chronic Obstructive Pulmonary Disease: Evidence from a Nationwide Prospective Cohort Study. *Environment & Health*. https://pubs.acs.org/doi/10.1021/envhealth.4c00198.

4. Bodur, M., et al. (2025). Immunomodulatory Effects of Omega-3 Fatty Acids: Mechanistic Insights and Health Implications. *Molecular Nutrition & Food Research*. https://onlinelibrary.wiley.com/doi/10.1002/mnfr.202400752.
5. Rudrapal, M., et al. (2022). Dietary Polyphenols and Their Role in Oxidative Stress-Induced Human Diseases: Insights into Protective Effects, Antioxidant Potentials and Mechanism(s) of Action. *Frontiers in Pharmacology*. https://www.frontiersin.org/journals/pharmacology/articles/10.3389/fphar.2022.806470/full.
6. Yahfoufi, N., et al. (2018). The Immunomodulatory and Anti-Inflammatory Role of Polyphenols. *Nutrients*. https://www.mdpi.com/2072-6643/10/11/1618.
7. Wibawa, J. C., et al. (2024). The Mechanism of Physical Exercise Increases Glutathione Peroxidase as an Endogenous Antioxidant: A Systematic Review. *Retos*. https://www.researchgate.net/publication/387583503_The_mechanism_of_physical_exercise_increases_glutathione_peroxidase_as_an_endogenous_antioxidant_a_systematic_review.
8. Hu, S., et al. (2023). Gut Microbial Beta-Glucuronidase: A Vital Regulator in Female Estrogen Metabolism. *Gut Microbes*. https://www.tandfonline.com/doi/full/10.1080/19490976.2023.2236749.
9. Collins, S. L., & Patterson, A. D. (2020). The Gut Microbiome: An Orchestrator of Xenobiotic Metabolism. *Acta Pharmaceutica Sinica B*. https://www.sciencedirect.com/science/article/pii/S2211383519309736?via%3Dihub.
10. Hodges, R. E., & Minich, D. M. (2015). Modulation of metabolic detoxification pathways using foods and food-derived components: A scientific review with clinical application. *Journal of Nutrition and Metabolism, 2015*, Article 760689. https://doi.org/10.1155/2015/760689.
11. Esteves, F., Rueff, J., & Kranendonk, M. (2021). The central role of cytochrome P450 in xenobiotic metabolism—A brief

review on a fascinating enzyme family. *Journal of Xenobiotics 11*(3), 94–114. https://doi.org/10.3390/jox11030007.
12. Calcium-D-glucarate (2002). *Alternative Medicine Review*, 7(4), 336–339. https://pubmed.ncbi.nlm.nih.gov/12197785.
13. Guengerich, F. P. (2008). Cytochrome p450 and Chemical Toxicology. *Chemical Research in Toxicology*. https://pubmed.ncbi.nlm.nih.gov/18052394/.
14. Hu, S., Ding, Q., Zhang, W., Kang, M., Ma, J., & Zhao, L. (2023). Gut microbial beta-glucuronidase: A vital regulator in female estrogen metabolism. *Gut Microbes*, *15*(1), Article 2236749. https://doi.org/10.1080/19490976.2023.2236749.

Chapter 11

Customize for Your Conditions and Life Stage

By now, you have identified your primary Hormone Type—Caretaker, Achiever, or Survivor—and have a better understanding of the beliefs, behavioral patterns, and imprinting that shape how your body responds to stress, nourishment, and daily life. You've learned about the importance of managing stress and anxiety, balancing your blood sugar, getting deep sleep, and other crucial components of your Hormone Action Plan. The core of your plan is in place. Now, it's time to fine-tune the plan based on specific conditions you may be experiencing, as well as the stage of life you are currently in.

In this chapter, I'll describe how I diagnose and develop a customized treatment plan for:

- Polyendocrine metabolic ovarian syndrome (PMOS)
- Endometriosis
- Metabolic syndrome
- Thyroid conditions

- PMS and PMDD
- Pregnancy and postpartum
- Perimenopause, menopause, and other estrogen-deficient groups

You Are Not Your Diagnosis

There's a reason why I have placed this chapter on specific conditions and life stages later in the book. Too often, women are taught to identify themselves by their diagnosis or their hormonal season. "I've got PMOS." "I'm a woman living with a chronic autoimmune disease." "I'm perimenopausal, so [eye roll, heavy sigh] *you know*. . ."

These labels can be helpful, but they are also incomplete, and they can sometimes become limiting, or even become a self-fulfilling prophecy. A diagnosis tells me where the hormonal imbalance shows up, not who you are and certainly not what you are capable of.

I caution my patients not to over-identify with any particular condition or stage of life. Remember that a diagnosis describes your present, not your future. Be mindful of the language you use to describe who you are. Because the words we say aloud repeatedly tend to become beliefs, which become behaviors, which become patterns, which lead to outcomes.

Consider the difference between these two statements:

> "I have a chronic condition that flares up and sometimes makes it difficult to function. It has negatively impacted every part of life, including my career and relationships. The flare-ups are unpredictable, and I'm always bracing myself for when the next one might arise."

> "I have a hormonal imbalance right now, and I'm taking steps to change this. It may take a while to restore balance, but already I'm noticing exciting changes that I can see reflected on my lab reports, and I can feel a difference too."

Both statements are accurate and truthful. Both statements could be made by the same women—someone experiencing severe endometriosis, for example. But these two statements carry a very different energy. The first sounds like a life sentence with no chance of parole. The second sounds like a temporary situation that can improve—and in fact, already is.

While it's important to consider your conditions and life stage and to refine your plan accordingly, don't lose sight of the bigger picture. What transforms outcomes is everything you've already learned to build: your rhythms, your daily habits, how you move and nourish, your sleep, your nervous system, your metabolic stability, and your detox support. That's the engine room of the ship. This chapter simply adjusts the sail.

As you read on, I will take you through the framework I use in my clinical practice to assess, diagnose, and treat some of the most common hormone-related conditions that women experience. You'll see how I approach these conditions and seasons of life and how I layer the evidence, physiology, and natural medicine tools to individualize care. I will also give my perspective on when to bring in pharmaceutical tools (including bioidentical hormone replacement therapy or medication to manage blood sugar levels) if that is something you and your healthcare team decide would be beneficial for your situation.

As we move through each scenario, I want you to keep these truths close:

You are not your diagnosis. You are not your life stage. You are the sum of your habits, your nourishment, your boundaries, and the consistency with which you honor your physiology.

I often think about this through the lens of an animal, because at the end of the day, that's what we are. If you take any animal and disrupt its basic biological needs: steady nourishment, predictable rhythms, movement, rest, detoxification, connection with its environment, connection with its circadian rhythm, or the protective structure of its community, that animal doesn't thrive. It struggles.

We see this in study after study on wildlife, on primates, even on domesticated animals: remove them from the conditions they're built for, and their physiology unravels. The same is true for us.

This is why I believe so deeply in naturopathic medicine. At the core of our philosophy is *Vis Medicatrix Naturae*: the body's instinctive capacity to heal when given the conditions it needs. Every therapy we choose, including medications or procedures, *if needed*, works best when it's layered onto a rich, nourished foundation rather than used as a stand-alone solution. Support the core first, and the higher-level interventions become more effective, more durable, and far less chaotic for the system. Strengthen the conditions, and the body will rise to meet you; skip them, and even the most advanced intervention has nowhere solid to land.

Once we cover the specific conditions and life stages, Chapter 12 will bring us back to the heart of this entire approach, the part too many women skip, the part no lab test will ever measure, and the part that determines whether your plan actually works: community, support, and belonging.

Polyendocrine Metabolic Ovarian Syndrome

Polyendocrine metabolic ovarian syndrome affects up to 15% of reproductive-aged women worldwide, yet it remains one of the most misunderstood and undertreated conditions in women's health.

PMOS is not simply a fertility issue or a period problem. It is a complex endocrine–metabolic condition sitting at the intersection of hormones, insulin signaling, inflammation, genetics, and environment. While medications such as hormonal contraceptives or metformin can be helpful in certain cases, they often address symptoms without fully correcting the underlying metabolic terrain driving the condition.

When untreated or undertreated, PMOS carries long-term risks beyond reproduction. Chronic insulin resistance, anovulation, and inflammation increase the risk of type 2 diabetes, cardiovascular disease, fatty liver disease, sleep apnea, and endometrial cancer. This is a whole-body condition with lifelong implications—which is why early, individualized intervention matters.

The encouraging reality is that when we address insulin regulation, inflammatory load, androgen excess, and hormonal rhythm, ovulation often returns, cycles regulate, skin clears, and long-term metabolic health improves. PMOS exists on a spectrum. Understanding the pattern is key.

The Four PMOS Phenotypes

Diagnostic guidelines (NIH, Rotterdam, AE-PMOS Society) describe four phenotypes. These represent variations of the same underlying physiology:

Phenotype A ("Classic PMOS")
Hyperandrogenism + ovulatory dysfunction + polycystic ovarian morphology.
Typically, the most metabolically affected.

Phenotype B
Hyperandrogenism + ovulatory dysfunction, without polycystic ovaries on imaging.

Phenotype C
Hyperandrogenism + polycystic ovaries, with regular ovulation.
Often seen in lean women with acne or hirsutism.

Phenotype D
Ovulatory dysfunction + polycystic ovaries, without elevated androgens.
Often milder metabolically.

Common symptoms across phenotypes include:

- Irregular or heavy periods
- Acne or oily skin
- Excess facial or body hair
- Hair thinning
- Weight gain or difficulty losing weight
- Mood changes
- Subfertility or anovulation

Phenotypes describe presentation. They do not explain the cause.

PMOS is highly individual, but the main root causes tend to cluster in seven domains:

1. **Genetics**
   Approximately 65–70% of cases have a genetic component affecting androgen production, LH signaling, insulin sensitivity, and follicle development. Genetics increase susceptibility—they do not eliminate agency.
2. **Hormonal Dysregulation**
   Elevated LH overstimulates ovarian theca cells, increasing androgen production.
   Insufficient FSH impairs follicle maturation.
   Elevated AMH keeps follicles in early development.
   The result is irregular ovulation and androgen excess.
3. **Insulin Resistance**
   Present in 50–70% of women with PMOS, regardless of body size. Elevated insulin stimulates ovarian androgen production and lowers SHBG, increasing free testosterone. For many women, this is the defining driver.
4. **Inflammatory Adiposity**
   Visceral fat functions as an inflammatory endocrine organ, worsening insulin resistance and hormonal imbalance. Body composition matters more than BMI.

5. **Environmental and Lifestyle Factors**
   Refined carbohydrates, endocrine-disrupting chemicals, chronic stress, and poor sleep amplify insulin resistance and inflammation.
6. **Adrenal Contribution**
   20–30% of women exhibit elevated DHEA-S, reflecting adrenal-driven androgen excess, often worsened by chronic stress.
7. **Medication-Induced Patterns**
   Certain medications can provoke a PMOS-like physiology by altering androgen or estrogen balance.

How PMOS Is Diagnosed

The Rotterdam criteria require two of the following three:

- Androgen excess (clinical or laboratory)
- Ovulatory dysfunction
- Polycystic ovarian morphology on ultrasound

Because PMOS overlaps with other endocrine disorders, evaluation should also exclude thyroid dysfunction, hyperprolactinemia, congenital adrenal hyperplasia, Cushing's syndrome, and androgen-secreting tumors.

My Approach: Restore Ovulation by Treating the Terrain

The fastest way to fail a PMOS treatment plan is to chase symptoms or supplements without addressing the broader terrain. That is why my framework always begins with these foundational steps. We want to improve:

- Blood sugar regulation
- Insulin sensitivity
- Inflammation and oxidative stress

- Androgen production and clearance
- Cortisol patterns and stress physiology
- Gut and liver function

When we stabilize the foundation, symptoms (and even PCOM, the small cysts on the ovaries) often resolve without forcing the ovaries with medications.

Dr. Dunlap's PMOS Approach

Scan to see my **PMOS Treatment Approach**—the strategies I use most often at my women's health clinic, including dietary changes, movement, evidence-supported supplements, and more.

Endometriosis

Endometriosis is not just a "painful period" condition. It is an estrogen-driven, immune-mediated inflammatory disease that disrupts pelvic, digestive, neurological, and hormonal systems. Lesions secrete inflammatory cytokines, recruit immune cells, and sensitize the central nervous system, creating a chronic pain loop that affects fertility, digestion, sleep, and mood.

Conventional therapies such as continuous hormonal contraceptives, progestins, NSAIDs, and GnRH analogs remain first-line for pain reduction and disease suppression, with surgery reserved for severe or refractory cases. But these modalities, if used alone, aren't necessarily addressing the whole-body complexity: the chronic inflammatory, immune, gut, and nervous-system imbalances that shape day-to-day quality of life. This is where an integrative approach matters, with conventional and naturopathic medicine working together as a coordinated team.

My Approach: Reduce Inflammation First (Core Driver of Pain)

When treating women with endometriosis, my priorities are:

- Lower systemic inflammation
- Support estrogen metabolism
- Target pain pathways and nervous system sensitization
- Reduce exposure to pesticides, plastics, and other endocrine disruptors
- Strengthen the immune system and improve whole-body resilience

Dr. Dunlap's Endometriosis Approach

Scan to see my **Endometriosis Treatment Approach**—the evidence-aligned approach I use most often with women in my practice. Includes recommendations to lower inflammation, upgrade your lifestyle, and other powerful actions you can take.

Endometriosis is not a single disease, and no two women respond to the same plan. Some improve most with gut repair, some with hormonal suppression, some with anti-inflammatory nutrition, and many with a combination. Treatment must evolve with symptom patterns, life stage, fertility goals, and pain physiology.

Metabolic Syndrome

Metabolic syndrome is not a single diagnosis but a constellation of many overlapping factors, including:

- Metabolic shifts (a change in how your body generates and uses energy)
- Abdominal adiposity (excess fat in the stomach region, surrounding internal organs)
- Elevated triglycerides (elevated levels of fat in your blood, which can increase your risk of heart disease, stroke, and other serious conditions)
- High blood pressure (forces your heart to work harder than it ought to, strains your body and also increases your risk of heart disease and stroke)
- Low HDL (high-density lipoprotein [HDL] is the "good cholesterol," the kind that helps reduce plaque build-up and clogged arteries)
- Elevated fasting glucose (significantly raises the risk of cardiovascular disease and type 2 diabetes)

For women, metabolic syndrome is particularly important because it often emerges silently and is deeply intertwined with hormonal transitions. In menopause, risk rises sharply as estrogen declines and abdominal fat, insulin resistance, and dyslipidemia increase. Women with PMOS, a history of gestational diabetes, chronic stress, lower socioeconomic support, or certain ethnic backgrounds (including South Asian, Indigenous, Hispanic, and non-Hispanic Black women) carry disproportionately higher risk.

The most critical piece many women are never told is that **adipose tissue is an endocrine organ—not inert storage**. Enlarged and inflamed fat cells release cytokines like IL-6 and TNF-α, elevate hs-CRP, and drive a chronic inflammatory state that disrupts insulin signaling, cortisol balance, cardiovascular health, and hormone metabolism.

And it's not the total amount of fat that matters most; it's *where* it's stored. Visceral fat (that's the kind of fat stored deep inside your body, surrounding your internal organs, hidden from view) acts like a metabolically "hot" endocrine organ, while subcutaneous fat (fat located close to your skin that you can grab or pinch) is far less risky. This is why BMI is such a poor tool for women; it cannot distinguish visceral fat from muscle, and many women with "normal" BMI carry the high-risk "skinny-fat" phenotype of low muscle and high visceral fat. Waist-to-hip ratio, visceral fat percentage, skeletal muscle mass, and metabolic biomarkers tell a far more accurate story.

My Approach: Focus on Blood Sugar Stabilization, First

In clinical practice, restoring metabolic health requires a whole-systems approach, leading with:

- Stabilizing blood sugar rhythms
- Improving insulin sensitivity
- Lowering inflammation
- Increasing muscle

Dr. Dunlap's Metabolic Syndrome Approach

Scan to see my **Metabolic Syndrome Approach**, including nutrition recommendations and medication options that you and your healthcare team might consider, if needed, including GLP-1 receptor agonists (commonly known by their brand names, including Ozempic, Wegovy, and Mounjaro). You'll also see how to mimic the benefits of these medications using natural, pharmaceutical-free alternatives.

With metabolic syndrome, as with any condition, whether you choose a pharmaceutical or nonpharmaceutical approach, work with an expert to individualize your care.

Thyroid Conditions

Thyroid disorders are among the most common hormone-related conditions affecting women, and they often sit quietly beneath symptoms like fatigue, weight changes, mood shifts, cycle irregularities, constipation, hair loss, and temperature dysregulation. Hypothyroidism, especially Hashimoto's thyroiditis, is the most prevalent, driven by a combination of genetics, autoimmunity, nutrient insufficiencies, chronic stress, and inflammation. Hashimoto's reflects an immune system that has lost tolerance and begun targeting thyroid tissue, gradually reducing its ability to produce T4 and T3.

Because thyroid hormones influence every cell in the body, metabolism, digestion, menstrual regularity, fertility, cognition, and cardiovascular function dysfunction can create a wide ripple effect across a woman's physiology.

My Approach: Lifestyle Changes First, Add Medication If Needed

My clinic supports many women with thyroid conditions with a whole-body approach. The thyroid responds remarkably well to foundational care. We want to focus on:

- Stable blood sugar
- Anti-inflammatory nutrition
- Stress reduction
- Optimized gut health (especially in women with autoimmune patterns)

Dr. Dunlap's Approach for Thyroid Conditions

Scan to see my **Approach for Thyroid Conditions**, including dietary and lifestyle modifications, targeted nutrients, botanicals, and supplements, and my thoughts on synthetic thyroid hormone medications such as levothyroxine.

PMS and PMDD

Premenstrual syndrome (PMS) and premenstrual dysphoric disorder (PMDD) are hormone-brain conditions driven by an abnormal sensitivity to normal luteal-phase hormonal shifts, especially progesterone metabolites and serotonin signaling changes.

PMS affects ~20–30% of women. Common symptoms include bloating, breast tenderness, fatigue, irritability, mood swings, acne, and food cravings brought on by a dip in serotonin. PMDD, a severe and debilitating form of PMS, affects 2–6% and can be profoundly impairing, with symptoms like intense anger or rage, profound depression, anxiety, feelings of hopelessness or worthlessness, even suicidal thoughts.

With PMS and PMDD, symptoms arise only in the luteal phase (that's the second half of the menstrual cycle, after ovulation, and before your period begins), resolve with menstruation, and do not occur during pregnancy, pre-menarche, or after menopause, highlighting that these conditions are not about high or low hormone levels but rather experienced with the change or shift in hormone levels.

My Approach: Add Positive Lifestyle Habits, Subtract Triggers That Worsen Luteal Instability

Dr. Dunlap's PMS and PMDD Approach

Scan to see my **PMS and PMDD Approach**, including nutrition, sleep, and supplements recommendations. Feeling irritable, experiencing rage or despair, feeling anxious or depressed is *not* your true self. Change is possible.

For women with moderate to severe PMDD, I will occasionally recommend incorporating medication into the plan. These can pair well with integrative care.

- SSRIs (continuous or luteal-phase dosing)
- MHT for anyone in early perimenopause stage
- Combined oral contraceptives (especially drospirenone-containing pills)
- GnRH agonists (for severe, refractory cases)

Pregnancy and Postpartum

Pregnancy and postpartum are two of the most profound hormone states a woman will ever experience. But these seasons also require very specific medical oversight and individualized care, which is why the full depth of pregnancy physiology is beyond the scope of this book—and rightly belongs in the hands of your obstetrician or midwife. Their role is central during pregnancy, when maternal health, fetal development, medication safety, and obstetric considerations must guide every decision.

What I want to acknowledge here is not pregnancy management itself, but the hormonal architecture: pregnancy is a state of extraordinary hormonal abundance, soaring estradiol, progesterone, and placental hormones, followed by one of the steepest hormonal drops in all human physiology. And it's the postpartum transition, not pregnancy, where women are most often left without adequate guidance, support, or a roadmap for recovery.

Postpartum is not a window of "bouncing back." It is a neuroendocrine recalibration: estrogen and progesterone fall sharply, prolactin rises, thyroid physiology becomes more vulnerable, metabolic demand increases, sleep fragments, stress can reach new heights, and nutrient depletion is common. These shifts alone can shape mood, energy, healing, weight regulation, milk supply, and emotional resilience.

My Approach: Be Proactive and Plan Ahead (Before the Baby Arrives)

In our conventional healthcare system, newborns and infants have a series of check-ups to make sure everything is going smoothly. The pediatrician regularly checks the baby's height, weight, head circumference, and asks lots of questions ("How many wet diapers per day?" "Is she sleeping through the night?" "Showing signs of crawling?") to ensure that everything is on track.

But when it comes to the mother's physical and emotional well-being? Often, nobody is checking in regularly or offering support. She is left to fend for herself, during one of the most demanding and vulnerable times in her life. Sure, mom might be handed the Edinburgh Postnatal Depression Scale (EPDS) at her six-week postpartum check up and asked to self-report if she feels depressed. But aside from that, many mothers are given this message: "Your baby is here! Congratulations. Good bye and good luck."

This is why I strongly encourage women to be proactive and create a postpartum wellness plan. Just as many women come up with an action plan to improve fertility and increase the likelihood of conception, it's important to have a postpartum wellness plan, too. The best time to develop this plan? Ideally, before the new baby arrives. Because it can be very challenging to map out your postpartum action plan when you're caring for a newborn, sleep-deprived, and (if a first-time parent) learning hundreds of new skills (swaddling, rocking, feeding, soothing. . .) while recovering from birth. Plan ahead for a stronger, smoother transition.

Dr. Dunlap's Postpartum Approach

Scan to see my **Postpartum Approach**, focusing on nutrition to fortify, hydrate, and soothe the body, recommended nutrients, botanicals, and supplements, and lab testing to identify commonly missed hormonal imbalances.

Perimenopause, Menopause and Other Estrogen-Deficient Groups

Menopause is one of the most significant hormone transitions a woman will go through, yet for decades it has been neglected, medicalized without context, or dismissed altogether. Estrogen, progesterone, and testosterone are not simply "reproductive hormones." They are metabolic, anti-inflammatory, neuroprotective, and vascular-protective hormones that impact every major system in the body. There is a reason I introduced them in Chapter 1 as part of our very important hormones (VIHs). When these hormones decline, whether gradually through perimenopause or abruptly in premature ovarian insufficiency, the shift reverberates through metabolism, mood, cognition, sleep, bone, musculoskeletal, and cardiovascular health.

Estrogen-Deficient Groups (Premenopausal)

Some women experience estrogen deficiency long before the menopausal transition, and for them, the stakes are even higher. Functional hypothalamic amenorrhea, often driven by chronic stress, under-eating, overtraining, or a combination of the three, is one of the most common causes of reproductive-age estrogen deficiency. Others are born with or develop conditions such as Turner syndrome or primary ovarian insufficiency, or experience medically induced suppression from chemotherapy, ovarian surgery, or long-term hormonal treatments. Even lifestyle factors such as low BMI, smoking, epilepsy, and severe psychosocial stress can accelerate ovarian aging and deplete estrogen earlier than expected.

Across all these groups, early or prolonged estrogen loss dramatically increases the lifetime risk of cardiovascular disease, osteoporosis, fractures, metabolic syndrome, diabetes, depression, and even cognitive decline. Women who lose estrogen before age 40, whether spontaneously or from medical causes, carry a significantly higher all-cause mortality risk if not treated appropriately. This is why early diagnosis, proactive monitoring, and timely hormonal restoration are critical. Estrogen is not merely a reproductive hormone; it is a vascular, skeletal, metabolic, and neuroprotective hormone. When it is missing in the decades it is meant to be present, the consequences echo across a woman's entire lifespan.

As estrogen drops, so does its protective influence on inflammation, brain function, vascular tone, and insulin sensitivity. This is why so many women experience rising abdominal weight, blood sugar instability, temperature dysregulation, mood changes, vaginal dryness, and sleep fragmentation during this transition. It's also why the risk of cardiovascular disease, metabolic syndrome, osteoporosis, and cognitive decline increases in the postmenopausal years. These are not random, they are physiologic consequences of losing a hormone that had been quietly supporting your body for decades.

Why Menopausal Hormone Therapy (MHT) Matters

Because premature estrogen decline is such a serious problem, this is also where menopausal hormone therapy becomes not only valuable but, in many cases essential. MHT, in my evidence-based naturopathic opinion, fits into the category of a preventative wellness strategy that can improve a woman's lifespan and health span.

Recent evidence, including what is meticulously presented in *Estrogen Matters* by Dr. Avrum Bluming and Dr. Carol Tavris, shows that for most healthy women, body-identical/bio-identical hormone therapy is not only safe but profoundly protective when started in the appropriate window.

The New Menopause by Dr. Mary Claire Haver echoes the same message: women deserve accurate information, individualized care, and the option to use hormones without fear-based narratives shaped by outdated interpretations of the Women's Health Initiative (WHI). (I highly recommend these resources if you are looking to dive deeper into this topic.)

When prescribed appropriately, MHT can improve vasomotor symptoms, protect bone density, improve metabolic health, support cognitive function, and enhance quality of life. And in the case of premature ovarian insufficiency (POI, a condition where ovaries stop functioning normally before age 40), early menopause, or surgical menopause, MHT isn't just helpful; it is the standard of care to protect heart, brain, and bone health for decades to come.

Layer the Foundation First, Add Meds If Needed

I've been safely prescribing MHT for more than a decade. Long before this current wave of menopause awareness, my clinic was already supporting thousands of women through perimenopause, menopause, and postmenopause with individualized, evidence-informed hormone therapy.

What I've learned is this: MHT works best when the foundation is strong—when stress levels are managed, blood sugar is balanced, sleep is supported, movement is specific to this stage of life, inflammation is lowered, the gut is functioning well, and stress physiology is addressed. Hormones do incredible work, but they go only so far in a system that is chronically depleted.

At the same time, hormone therapy is not for everyone, and not every woman wants it. The North American Menopause Society (NAMS) outlines clear situations where MHT should be approached more cautiously, including in the presence of unexplained vaginal bleeding, active liver disease, estrogen-sensitive cancers, or recent cardiovascular events. These situations require thoughtful, expert-guided care. This is why partnering with a menopause-trained clinician is important. Proper evaluation, shared decision-making, and ongoing monitoring are critical.

My Approach: Mind-Body Medicine—Tailored to Midlife

Menopause is not a moment or a condition; it is a long hormonal transition with profound effects on the brain, heart, metabolism, bones, sleep, and emotional resilience. The goal here is to protect the systems most impacted by estrogen, progesterone, and testosterone decline while supporting women through the symptomatic changes of this transition and supporting their ongoing health span.

When I'm designing a treatment approach for perimenopause/menopause/postmenopause and other estrogen-deficient groups, the priorities are to:

- Reduce inflammation, regulate blood sugar, and protect cardiovascular health
- Preserve muscle/bone health and metabolic flexibility
- Use supplements as needed to buffer against the physiologic vulnerabilities that emerge during this transition
- Add in medication (menopausal hormone therapy [MHT]) where appropriate to help replace what's declining

Dr. Dunlap's Perimenopause/Menopause/ Postmenopause Approach

Scan the code to see my **Perimenopause/Menopause/ Postmenopause Approach**, which I use every day in my clinic for women experiencing perimenopause, menopause, postmenopause, and POI (premature recommendations regarding body-identical hormones such as estradiol, micronized progesterone, and testosterone therapy).

As always, discuss your approach with your naturopathic physician or another trusted healthcare provider and individualize the plan to your needs.

Treatment Plans Are for Human Beings—Not Just for Conditions

As a naturopathic physician, my approach is to develop a treatment plan for the *woman* sitting in front of me—rather than only developing a plan for her diagnosis, condition, or stage of life. While the latter informs the plan, I know she is much more than these.

Two women may come into my clinic, both with PMOS, painful PMS, a thyroid condition, or estrogen deficiency, yet the two women might be very different human beings. Different beliefs. Different behavioral patterns. Different goals. Different stressors and pressures in their lives. Different numbers on their lab reports, revealing different imbalances and providing different clues.

Sending both women out of my office with identical (or, almost identical) wellness plans would be doing them a great disservice. Yet unfortunately, this is what happens in many healthcare settings. Women are sent on their way with a generic two-page pamphlet ("Get the Facts on Blood Sugar") or with a prescription in hand, along with, "Let's get you back in here in six months to see how you're doing." This is not sufficient care. Not even close.

We are alike in many ways. At the same time, no two women are identical. Treatment plans should never be one-size-fits-all or even one-size-fits-most. And plans should never be static. They should constantly be evolving. There should be an initial plan, then follow-up testing and monitoring, and then adjustments to the plan as needed.

My hope is that you feel hopeful about the possibilities available to you, inspired to speak with your healthcare team about your options, and determined to customize your Hormone Action Plan to meet your exact needs.

Please don't copy-paste any of the approaches I present in the chapter and use it verbatim. These aren't protocols; these are ideas. Instead, use the methods I present as a jumping-off point for a conversation with your providers. While there are universal principles that inform most plans, the details must always be fine-tuned to the individual.

You deserve exceptional care in every season of your life. Please don't settle for anything less.

Key Takeaways

- You are more than your condition or life stage. Be mindful about the words you choose to describe yourself and try to avoid over-identifying with a diagnosis. Words become beliefs, and beliefs drive behavior and outcomes.
- While higher-level interventions (such as medication) can be helpful in some cases, it's important to build the foundation—including lifestyle changes, stress management, sleep, nutrition, movement, and supplements as needed.
- If you choose to include medication in your wellness plan, you'll have much better results once the foundation has been laid first. Where hormones are deficient, replacement (where appropriate) is also considered foundational.
- Developing a treatment plan should never be a quick copy-paste job. A woman's beliefs, behavioral patterns, family structure, sources of stress, personal challenges, the season of life she is in—all of this must be factored into the plan.
- Allow your plan to evolve. Do follow-up lab testing, monitor how symptoms are improving or worsening, have ongoing conversations with your providers, and adjust the plan accordingly.
- Although it is not always easy to get it, you deserve high-quality care. Fight for it. Because the end results—balanced hormones, a body that is functioning optimally, and radiant health—are worth the effort.

Key Takeaways

Chapter 12

Create Your Support Network

In Okinawa, Japan, there is an ancient tradition that has endured for centuries. When a child is born, she is assigned a special group of friends; they are companions who will stand by her side and show up in her time of need, all the days of her life. This group is called a *moai.*

A moai usually consists of five or six friends. As children, they meet regularly to play and make a pledge to support each other for a lifetime. As adults, they meet up frequently (once or twice a week, sometimes more) and strengthen each other's lives in different ways.

When one is sick, the others bring soup, tea, or healing herbs. When someone wants to buy a house, the others chip in to help cover the costs. When one loses their spouse, the others provide comfort during their time of grief.

Members of a moai meet up for walks, meals, or to simply talk about life. For the people of Okinawa, your moai is considered your second family. Sacred relationships. Worth more than gold.

In many industrialized countries, including the United States, centenarians—people who live to be 100 years of age or more—are quite rare. Just 10 to 20 centenarians per 100,000 adults,[1] sometimes up to 24 per 100,000[2] depending on the year, according to US Census reports. But Okinawa has "more than three times the numbers found in US populations of the same size," reports the BBC.[3]

In Okinawa, people not only live longer (7–10 years longer than Americans, on average) but are also less likely to suffer from illnesses that erode their quality of life. Their lifespan is longer. Their health span—the number of years lived in good health, free from disease—is longer, too.

Okinawans understand that your *support network* has a profound impact on the length and quality of your life, for several reasons. One, your community keeps you on track when it comes to sticking with healthy habits. Two, you need people who will swiftly come to your aid during times when you are vulnerable, sick, or stressed. And three, close relationships are emotionally rewarding—they're what make life worth living.

We Create Each Other, We Sustain Each Other

Okinawans aren't the only people who understand the life-changing, life-saving, and life-extending importance of social connection.

In Southern Africa, communities hold friendship circles rooted in the philosophy of *Ubuntu*: "I am because we are." Key tenets of the Ubuntu philosophy include the ideas that nobody can survive in isolation and that individual wellness is the shared responsibility of the collective.

"Ubuntu is a deep and embodied understanding that human beings are not born but formed in community and relationship with one another," write Pamela Ayo Yetunde, Rehena Harilall, Nobantu Mpotulo, David W. Robinson-Morris, and Yao Obiora Dibia in a collaborative article that they co-authored. "Our humanity is a collective endeavor; we create each other and sustain one another."[4]

In Bhutan, small groups meet for tea, song, and storytelling. Bhutan's 4th King, Jigme Singye Wangchuck, famously coined the term "Gross National Happiness" to describe Bhutan's focus on pursuing positive relationships and well-being rather than purely economic pursuits.[5]

Compadrazgo, a concept originating in Latin America with Catholic roots, means "shared parenthood." It's a tradition of spiritual kinship between the parents and godparents of a child.[6] A similar size group to the Okinawan moai, the compadrazgo typically includes five people: two parents, two godparents, and the child. *Compadres* become lifelong allies, supporting each other in joy, grief, and major life events, including graduations and quinceañeras, the Latin American celebration marking a girl's transition to womanhood when she turns 15.

Joseph Feldman, section editor for the Society for Latin American and Caribbean Anthropology, describes these Compadrazgo relationships as "kinship by choice"[7] rather than by blood. They are your chosen family.

The word *clachan* comes from a Gaelic term meaning stone, signifying a stone circle or settlement where people gather. Throughout Scotland and Ireland, clachans are tight-knit communities. Visiting neighbors, gathering to chat around the fire, and celebratory feasts are different ways to keep the clachan strong. Modern-day clachans meet up for "conversation, laughter, and plenty of storytelling," enjoying "gatherings that celebrate tradition, connection, and good cheer."[8] That's from a 2025 blog post from the Society of Old Friends, a UK organization that provides "a chance to reconnect, meet new people, and build lasting relationships."[9]

And in India, a *sangha* is a spiritual community of friends who are committed to walking the path of mindfulness together. Sangha means "assembly," "association," or "community," and the term can be used in a religious sense (ordained monks or nuns who live by a spiritual code) or nonreligious, referring to friends who gather to meditate, share joys and difficulties, and navigate life together.

In the Buddhist tradition, spending time with your sangha is akin to visiting a sanctuary—a place of refuge[10] where you can step away from the strain of the outside world, take off your armor, and receive support. Describing the value of these connections, Ernestine Enomoto writes, "We need only a committed group of ordinary people to receive great benefit from it [...] In a sangha, there is mutual helping. When we fall down, there is always someone who can help us up."

The Greatest Predictor of Well-Being: Connection

Whether you call it a moai, compadrazgo, clachan, sangha, or any other term, we all need a sacred circle of support.

Can you imagine how different your life would be, if you had one?

No matter where you live—a village in Bhutan or a suburb near Boise, Idaho—you can create a support network that enriches your life, enhances your health, and changes your future.

What I've found, after serving thousands of patients, is that social connection has a far greater impact on health outcomes than many of us think. Once you have a support network in place, everything else—managing stress and anxiety, balancing blood sugar, movement, diet, sleep—becomes more doable.

If you want to create a Hormone Action Plan and stick with it, long term, the largest factor that determines your success is your support network. This is why, in Figure 12.1, I put *Create Your Support Network* right in the center.

Connection needs to be a major focus, not an afterthought. This is the beating heart that powers every other part of your plan.

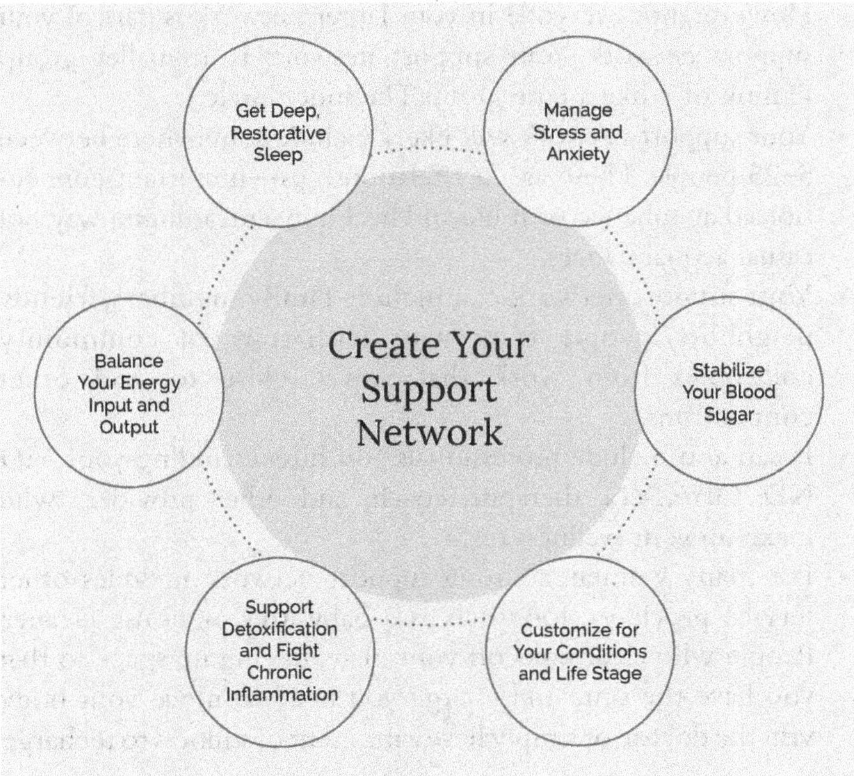

Figure 12.1 Your Hormone Action Plan.

What Is a Support Network?

I've used the phrase *support network* numerous times in the chapter, but what does this actually mean? Here's how I define it:

- Your support network is a group of people who help you to become the healthiest, most flourishing version of yourself.
- Your larger personal and/or professional network may include 150 people or more. (British anthropologist Robin Dunbar theorizes that most people can sustain only around 150 relationships at most.[11])

- However, not everyone in your larger network is part of your support network. Your support network is a smaller group. (Think of it like a core group. The inner circle.)
- Your support network will likely include somewhere between 5–25 people. These are key relationships—important connections that enhance your life and health in a meaningful way, not casual acquaintances.
- Your support network can include family members, friends, neighbors, people from your faith/spiritual community, colleagues from work that you're close to, and other connections.
- It can also include professionals you hire, including your MD, ND, OB/GYN, therapist, coach, and other providers who make up your wellness team.
- For many women, a strong support network includes other service providers, too, such as a babysitter or house cleaner. People who clear tasks off your plate, freeing up space so that you have the time and energy you need to move your body, visit the doctor, or simply have a moment of stillness to recharge.

Three Categories of Support

When creating your support network, the three main categories to think about are *emotional support* (this can include your spouse or partner, family, friends, neighbors, people in your book club or from yoga class), *expert support* (your physician, naturopathic doctor, gynecologist, a wellness coach, etc.), and *helper support* (babysitter, housekeeper, or personal assistant who handles errands).

Ideally, your network will include all three—emotional, expert, and helper—so that it is strong and well-rounded. Each of these relationships will be unique and have different levels of intimacy (you may not confide in your babysitter the same way you do with your best friend), but they are all powerful additions to your network and contribute to your health in important ways.

Every woman's support network looks a bit different. The common denominator is this: these are people who help you move closer to a 10 on the Wellness Spectrum, rather than dragging you down towards a 0.

Why Does This Matter?

Connection is medicine. The relationships in your life have a direct impact on all the systems in your body—yes, including your endocrine system, the one responsible for hormone production. Numerous studies confirm the connection between having a strong support network and increasing both lifespan and health span. Lack of connection can have disastrous consequences:

- **The Harvard Nurses' Health Study**[12]
  Researchers tracked 72,000 women for 22 years. Those who were socially connected lived 10% longer and were 41% more likely to reach age 85 or older, compared to women who led more isolated lives.
- **Loneliness and Social Isolation as Risk Factors for Mortality: A Meta-Analytic Review**[13]
  In this study, published in *Perspectives on Psychological Science*, researchers found that loneliness, isolation, and living alone increased risk of death by 26–32%. Their findings show that disconnection from others is just as detrimental to your health as obesity or leading a sedentary lifestyle.

On the other side of the coin, social connection can boost your well-being in remarkable ways:

- **Study on Exercise Contagion in a Global Social Network**[14]
  This study, involving 1.1 million runners, shows that when your friend decides to run an extra kilometer (0.62 miles), you are likely to run farther than you otherwise would. An extra 0.3 kilometers on average. Putting in extra effort is contagious.

- **Partner Influence in Diet and Exercise Behaviors: Testing Behavior Modeling, Social Control, and Normative Body Size**[15]
  Published in the *PLOS One* journal from the Public Library of Science, this study found that when one person in a married or cohabitating couple chooses to change their diet or exercise routine, their partner is likely to change too—a 13–20% effect in behavior change. Researchers say, "Adoption of exercise or diet modifications in one individual is likely to spread to others, creating a social environment characterized by mutual reinforcement of healthy behavior."

  Bringing health-conscious people into your life—your spouse or partner, family, friends, colleagues—can positively influence your habits and health.

Research also shows that having a multidisciplinary healthcare team—rather than just one provider—also leads to improved patient outcomes.

- **Collaborative Care for Women with Depression: A Systematic Review**[16]
  This review analyzed seven articles from medical journals to look for common themes. Their findings: women with depression are more likely to improve when they have a team that combines physicians, mental health professionals, and other providers, rather than "just" a physician or therapist.
- **The Effect of Multidisciplinary Team on Survival Rates of Women with Breast Cancer: A Systematic Review and Meta-Analysis**[17]
  "Breast cancer is the seventh-highest cause of cancer deaths globally," report the team behind this review. However, a woman is more likely to survive when she has a multidisciplinary team, which can include her physician, oncologist, surgeon, genetic counselors, social workers, and other providers.

An integrated approach leads to better outcomes, especially when the various team members discuss their overall strategy through "well-organized MDT discussions." (MDT stands for multidisciplinary team.)

When providers put their brains together, they achieve results that no single person could ever reach alone. That's one of the reasons why my women's health clinic, Naturopathic By Design, has a team of 10 providers including licensed naturopathic doctors, registered nurses, and functional nutritionists.

I could include 100+ more pages detailing the copious amounts of scientific research, but I know you're already seeing the point: having a support network will improve and lengthen your life.

This is why creating your support network is the center of your Hormone Action Plan.

It is extremely difficult to achieve optimal health when you're trying to do it alone, or perhaps with one doctor or one therapist helping you. This just isn't enough support. It is much easier to manage stress and anxiety, eat well, move well, sleep well, and keep your hormones in balance when you have a well-rounded support network in place.

How to Create Your Support Network

So many of the women I work with understand the importance of having a strong support network and truly want to create one. But the main obstacles are lack of time and energy.

"I'm already so busy. Creating a support network feels like 'yet another thing' I have fit into my life."

"I don't have energy to build new relationships."

"I barely have enough energy to pay attention to the relationships I already have."

"It's hard to meet people as an adult, especially if you live in an isolated area/work from home/don't go out much/etc."

Here's a reframe: what if creating your support network was energy-giving, rather than energy-draining? What if these relationships could create more free time and open space in your life, rather than less? And what if curating your network could be simpler and less daunting than you think?

Here are my tips on how to create a well-rounded support network—one that includes emotional support, expert support, and helper support—even if you have the busiest life imaginable:

- **Evaluate your current network**
  Make a list of the people who provide emotional support, expert support, and helper support in your life right now. Remember, this list can include family, friends, neighbors, colleagues, healthcare providers, domestic or childcare helpers, and others. You might end up with a list of 5–25 people—or more! Your support network may already be larger than you think. (Perhaps you don't need to go out and build new relationships, but rather, tap into the ones you already have.)
- **Identify who is missing**
  As you review your list, where are the gaps? Maybe your list includes great friends but few people on your healthcare team. Or perhaps you have wonderful connections, but they all live in other cities, and you need more local support. Consider, "Who could I bring into my support network so that it is stronger and more well-rounded?"
- **Initiate *one* new connection**
  Once you have identified who is missing, take one proactive step to bring that person into your network. This could mean booking a consultation with a new healthcare provider or RSVPing for an event where you're likely to meet some new people in your local area, or another step. You don't have to construct your entire support network today. Start with one new relationship.

- **Deepen *one* existing connection**
  Is there a friend or family member whom you love but haven't reached out to in a while? Send a text or voice note or call to check in. Strengthen one connection that you already have.
- **Invite someone to join for an activity you're already doing**
  If your Hormone Action Plan includes taking a daily walk, invite someone to join you. If you want to learn new practices for nervous system regulation and you're considering taking a class, invite a friend to come. You can incorporate connection into your daily rhythm without making it an "extra" thing you have to do.
- **Choose forms of connection that fill your energy tank**
  Especially if you are introverted, going to a bustling dinner party with 15 people talking across the table in a loud restaurant may not feel good! Instead, choose options that work for your personality. This can look like calling a friend and chatting while you do meal prep or scheduling a playdate for the kids while you enjoy a cup of tea and conversation with another mom. Connection can be peaceful, rejuvenating, and quiet—if that's what you prefer.
- **Systematize your support network**
  When you schedule things in advance, it's less mentally taxing to build and nurture your network. For instance, schedule your weekly walk with a friend, schedule your bi-weekly check in with your naturopathic physician, schedule your monthly book club night—in advance. Set it up on your calendar as a recurring appointment and then you can put it out of your mind. By doing this, you'll connect with important people from your network automatically without having to remember. "Past You" already set up the system so that "Present You" can enjoy the benefits.

- **Embrace quality over quantity**
  You may have a treasured girlfriend that you see only once a year on your annual weekend trip. Even if it's "only" two days together, make this time count. A short visit with them can fill up your connection tank more than dozens of rushed, frantic appointments.
- **Hiring service providers counts**
  Depending on what phase of life you are in, adding helper support to your network may be the most powerful move you can make. A babysitter, nanny, housekeeper, or local college student who helps with errands can be a life-altering investment in your health. You don't necessarily need to hire full-time salaried help, but maybe a few hours a week would offer relief and fit your budget. If someone handles laundry, for instance, this could bring you three extra hours a week[18] that you can put toward fitness, nutrition, sleep, or building quality connections with others in your network.

As you take steps to build your support network, share your Hormone Action Plan with one or two women that you love and trust. Tell them what you've learned from this book and how you've been putting together your personalized plan. Invite them to create their own plans and join you on the journey toward flourishing health.

You can form your own wellness group with one or two women who share your goals, meeting up for walks or meals and sharing wisdom and resources ("I just found the *best* chiropractor. . .") and solidarity. Perhaps in time, your group can grow.

Let Them Know You

When Vanessa Cornell—Harvard graduate, mom of five, and founder of the wellness brand NUSHU—was 35 years old, her husband said, "Vanessa, you don't have any friends."

Hearing this, Vanessa felt defensive. She describes what happened next on a podcast interview with host Katie Fogarty.[19]

"What are you talking about?" she replied to her husband.

He insisted, "You don't share anything with anybody. You don't confide in people."

These words stung but also created a moment of awakening for Vanessa. As much as it pained her to admit it, she realized he was right.

She had been operating under the assumption that the way to build strong relationships was to show others the most "perfect" and "appealing" version of yourself: the version of you that is poised, polished, successful, and confident even when that's not how she felt. Although she knew a lot of wonderful women, she didn't feel particularly close to anyone because she had never allowed anyone to truly *know* her.

Something shifted inside of Vanessa that day. She decided, "I am going to tell the truth about myself out loud, as ugly as it is, to as many people as possible."

She began sharing the messier parts of her life with women she knew—her marriage troubles, insecurities, and other things she had previously kept hidden. When she shared more of herself, women weren't repulsed. They didn't abandon her; they leaned in.

They said, "I feel the same way" or "I've been there, too." They shared their own stories. Gradually, some of Vanessa's distant acquaintances became close friends—her chosen family.

Vulnerability was the piece that had been missing all along—and it's what allowed her to create the support network she wanted and needed. (After watching a documentary series about longevity, Vanessa became fascinated with the Okinawan concept of a moai and couldn't stop thinking about it. She described the Okinawan tradition to a mutual colleague of ours, Alexandra, who then told me about it a few months later. Wisdom shared—one woman to another. Today, Vanessa's mission is to help every woman create her own modern-day moai, which she helps to facilitate through events, retreats, and her podcast, *Voicenotes from a Friend*.)

When you're dealing with something challenging—a painful health condition, an overwhelming work schedule, issues with your spouse, or anything else—you may feel compelled to keep quiet and hide what's happening. You think, "I don't want to complain or be a burden to others." But when you pretend like "everything is fine" (when it's not), as Vanessa learned, you build walls between yourself and others. Silence makes your support network weaker, not stronger.

There are people who would genuinely love to support you—if given the chance. But first, you have to open up. People can't offer support if they have no idea what you're going through or what you need.

Be a Villager

If you are thinking that it sounds like a lot of work to build a support network, you're not wrong. It is. But it can be joyful, meaningful work—not drudgery.

Writer Candice McClue says, "Everyone wants a village, but no one wants to be a villager." There's truth to this statement. Many women wish they had a village of tight-knit friends, relatives, neighbors, and other connections, but many of us resist the effort to build these life-affirming connections.

Being a villager means checking on a friend who is going through a hard time. Signing up for the meal train when a neighbor is having a baby. Offering to drive a colleague to their healthcare appointment. Taking the initiative to plan gatherings to bring people together. Telling your friends about your favorite physician, naturopathic doctor, doula, or midwife, and posting a five-star review on that provider's site to support their work. The effort doesn't have to (and shouldn't) fall solely on your shoulders, but you do need to do your part as a villager.

Yes, it takes effort—*connect* is a verb—but this is what creating your moai, clachan, or sangha requires. The benefits are worth the effort you put in. These are the actions that improve your quality of life immediately and that can add another 10 years to your lifespan and health span in the future.

Specific Recommendations for the Caretaker, Achiever, and Survivor

No matter your Hormone Type, you need strong support in your life. But, depending on your type, you may have certain beliefs, behaviors, and patterns that stop you from getting the support you need and want. The following are a few suggestions tailored to each type.

The Caregiver

Your Pattern: Because you are stretched thin caring for everyone else, your nervous system rarely experiences true relief. You protect, organize, anticipate, and manage—often without receiving equal support in return. The very thing that would create the greatest hormonal shift for you is the thing you resist most: allowing others to carry more.

Your first step is increasing helper support so your system can downshift from chronic output to restoration.

Your Three Highest-Leverage Moves

1. **Increase practical support.**
   Ask your partner to take on defined responsibilities. Hire help where possible. Create creative exchanges if needed.
2. **Reclaim time for actual restoration.**
   If you secure childcare or assistance, use that time for recovery, not productivity. Rest, move gently, sit in silence, or do something that fills you instead of drains you.
3. **Affirmation:**
   "I give help generously and consistently to others. I need and deserve help, too."

The Achiever

Your Pattern: You excel at structure, optimization, and external support. Your calendar is full, your goals are clear, and your network likely includes trainers, coaches, and professionals. What is often undernourished is emotional connection.

When relationships receive only your leftover energy, imbalance quietly builds.

Your Three Highest-Leverage Moves

1. **Schedule memory-making experiences.**
   Take a day off work and play hooky with your kids, schedule a spa day for you and your spouse.
2. **Invest in emotional depth.**
   Slow down enough to know your neighbor's name. Linger in conversation. Replace efficiency with presence. Plan a weekend getaway with loved ones.
3. **Affirmation:**
   "Success is not just how much I accomplish. It's also measured in the depth and strength of my most important relationships."

The Survivor

Your Pattern: You have endured significant stress—emotionally, physically, or environmentally—and your system carries the imprint. Your health story is often layered and complex. Quick fixes have likely failed you before.

What you need most are safety, consistency, and a team that sees the full picture.

Your Three Highest-Leverage Moves

1. **Build a multidisciplinary power team.**
   Seek providers who listen deeply, investigate thoroughly, and collaborate rather than prescribe reflexively. Avoid rushed, surface-level care.

2. **Curate your environment.**
   Spend time around people whose energy is expansive, hopeful, and forward-moving. Stagnation reinforces stress physiology, but vitality is contagious.
3. **Affirmation:**
   "I surround myself with vibrant, life-giving people who strengthen my health and future."

Creating My Circle of Support

I don't live on the island of Okinawa or in a remote village in Bhutan. Nevertheless, I have created my own sacred circle of support. This includes emotional support, expert support, and helper support—in many forms. My support network has come into existence because of intentional decisions.

My husband and I chose to move to Portland, Maine, because it would mean being closer to our daughters' grandparents and creating more support in our lives.

I chose to expand my team at the clinic, growing from one provider—me—to a team of more than 10 women. I knew I couldn't achieve my goal of impacting thousands of women alone.

I have cultivated relationships with remarkable friends and colleagues—many of whom offered their support so generously while I was writing this book. Several chapters were written at a friend's beach house. Other chapters, at another friend's mountain cabin. They recognized how much this project meant to me and that I needed silence and solitude to get it done—and they stepped in to help.

Building my support network didn't happen all at once. It was woven together, one connection at a time. There have been times in my life when my network felt weaker, but little by little, through deliberate action, one relationship at a time, it has grown stronger.

"The relationships you're cultivating right now will dictate what you're achieving one, five, or ten years down the line," writes

Selena Soo,[20] a colleague and author of the *USA Today* bestseller *Rich Relationships*. Soo is primarily talking about relationships that help you achieve professional goals, but her message applies to wellness goals too. If your goal is to restore hormonal balance and achieve flourishing health, having the right people in your circle will make all the difference.

Who is one treasured person you already have in your network? How could you pour more energy into this connection to make it even stronger? Start with one person. It can be someone you already know.

You may already be connected to incredible people who would love to play a bigger role in your life—if you let them. Just as you long to have more support, they do too. You will create it together.

Key Takeaways

- Research shows that people with a strong support network live longer, are healthier, experience less disease overall, and are more likely to survive serious diseases (including breast cancer) if one should happen.
- Building a support network isn't optional—it's preventive medicine that changes your lifespan and health span.
- Many cultures around the world—from Okinawa to Bhutan and beyond—understand that social connection is essential for well-being and must be prioritized.
- A strong support network includes *emotional support* (friends, family, and neighbors who uplift you), *expert support* (health and wellness professionals), and *helper support* (practical support such as childcare, cleaning, or assistance with daily tasks).

- Having all three types of support in your network creates stability and strength, helping you sustain healthy habits and handle the demands of your life without burning out.
- It's important to remember that having a village means being a villager—giving support as well as receiving.
- If you don't feel as close to others as you wish you did, consider, *Am I letting people truly know me?* Take off your armor, share some of the messier parts of your life, and often, others will do the same. Vulnerability can close the emotional distance and solidify your bond.
- Building your support network doesn't happen overnight. It takes time. Even just one connection can make such a difference. Start with one relationship and expand from there.

Notes

1. Willcox, D. C., et al. (2006). Genetic Determinants of Exceptional Human Longevity: Insights from the Okinawa Centenarian Study. *Age (Dordr).* https://pmc.ncbi.nlm.nih.gov/articles/PMC3259160/.
2. "United States Census Bureau." Release dated Monday, September 22, 2025. https://www.census.gov/newsroom/press-releases/2025/centenarian-population.html.
3. "A High-Carb Diet May Explain Why Okinawans Live So Long." BBC. Robson, D. 2019. https://www.bbc.com/future/article/20190116-a-high-carb-diet-may-explain-why-okinawans-live-so-long.
4. "Ubuntu: I Am Because We Are." Lion's Roar. Yetunde, P. A., et al. 2022. https://www.lionsroar.com/ubuntu-i-am-because-we-are/.

5. "Bhutan's Gross National Happiness (GNH) Index." OECD. OECD. 2024. https://www.oecd.org/en/publications/well-being-knowledge-exchange-platform-kep_93d45d63-en/bhutan-s-gross-national-happiness-gnh-index_ff75e0a9-en.html.
6. "The Continuing Relevance of Compadrazgo Spiritual Kinship in Latin America." Anthropology News. Alum, R. A. 2024. https://www.anthropology-news.org/articles/the-continuing-relevance-of-compadrazgo-spiritual-kinship-in-latin-america/.
7. "The Continuing Relevance of Compadrazgo Spiritual Kinship in Latin America." Anthropology News. Alum, R. A. 2024. https://www.anthropology-news.org/articles/the-continuing-relevance-of-compadrazgo-spiritual-kinship-in-latin-america/.
8. "2025 Summer Clachan, Manchester." The Society of Old Friends. The Society of Old Friends. 2025. https://thesocietyofoldfriends.co.uk/2025-summer-clachan-manchester/.
9. "The Society of Old Friends." The Society of Old Friends. 1909. https://thesocietyofoldfriends.co.uk/.
10. "Nourished and Sustained by Sangha." Still Water Mindfulness Practice Center. Still Water MPC. 2018. https://www.stillwatermpc.org/dharma-topics/nourished-and-sustained-by-sangha/.
11. "Dunbar's Number: Why We Can Only Maintain 150 Relationships." BBC Future. Dunbar, R. 2019. https://www.bbc.com/future/article/20191001-dunbars-number-why-we-can-only-maintain-150-relationships.
12. Trudel-Fitzgerald, C., et al. (2020). The Prospective Association of Social Integration with Life Span and Exceptional Longevity in Women. *The Journals of Gerontology: Series B, Psychological Sciences & Social Sciences.* https://pubmed.ncbi.nlm.nih.gov/31495897/.

13. Holt-Lunstad, J., et al. (2015). Loneliness and Social Isolation as Risk Factors for Mortality: A Meta-Analytic Review. *Perspectives on Psychological Science*. https://journals.sagepub.com/doi/abs/10.1177/1745691614568352.
14. Eagle, N., et al. (2017). Exercise Contagion in a Global Social Network. *Nature Communications*. https://www.nature.com/articles/ncomms14753.
15. Perry, B., et al. (2016). Partner Influence in Diet and Exercise Behaviors: Testing Behavior Modeling, Social Control, and Normative Body Size. *PLOS ONE*. https://journals.plos.org/plosone/article?id=10.1371/journal.pone.0169193.
16. Huang, H., et al. (2017). Collaborative Care for Women with Depression. *Psychosomatics*. https://pubmed.ncbi.nlm.nih.gov/27842779/.
17. Pangarsa, E. A., et al. (2023). The Effect of Multidisciplinary Team on Survival Rates of Women with Breast Cancer: A Systematic Review and Meta-Analysis. *Annals of Medicine and Surgery (London)*. https://pubmed.ncbi.nlm.nih.gov/37363480/.
18. "How Much Time Do Wash and Fold Laundry Services Really Save You?" Top Wash Laundry. Top Wash Laundry. 2024. https://topwashlaundry.com/how-much-time-do-wash-and-fold-laundry-services-really-save-you/#.
19. "Vanessa Cornell on the Transformative Power of Female Friendship at Midlife." A Certain Age. Fogarty, K., & Cornell, V. 2025. https://www.acertainagepod.com/shows/vanessa-cornell-on-the-transformative-power-of-female-friendship-at-midlife.
20. Soo, S. Facebook post dated October 13, 2025. https://www.facebook.com/SelenaSoo/photos/you-may-not-see-the-impact-of-your-relationships-right-away-but-years-later-they/1344197220395490/.

Bringing It All Together: Three Sample Plans

If you've made it to this point, well done! By now. . .

You've Got a Solid Education About Your Body

You've been introduced to your body's 50+ hormones and understand the important functions they perform. You may feel a sense of gratitude and awe for your hormones (I often call them "sacred chemical messengers") and everything they do. And, you've learned the factors that cause hormones to get out of whack, from chronic stress to poor sleep to environmental toxins and beyond.

You Know Your Hormone Type

Caretaker. Achiever. Survivor. These aren't labels. They're lenses. Each one helps reveal the behavioral patterns, stress signatures, and energetic tendencies that shape your physiology. You now understand the "why" behind your symptoms, not just the "what."

You Understand the Seven Components of Your Hormone Action Plan

A plan that focuses on "just one thing" (such as supplements or medication) doesn't work. That's why your Hormone Action Plan includes seven components, not one. All the layers of your plan work together to shift your physiology. You've learned how to:

- Manage stress and anxiety
- Stabilize your blood sugar
- Get deep, restorative sleep
- Balance your energy input and output
- Support detoxification and fight chronic inflammation
- Customize for your conditions and life stage
- Create your support network

And now for the final step, the part where theory becomes action, and action becomes transformation.

Three Sample Plans

To bring it all together, I have created three sample plans for you—one for each Hormone Type.

Scan to download three sample **Hormone Action Plans**—a plan for the Caretaker, Achiever, and Survivor.

How the Sample Plans Are Structured

For each sample plan, I provide a **Personalized Prescription** that includes detailed information on lab tests to be performed, dietary and lifestyle changes, supplements, and more.

After this, you'll see a section called **Your First 30 Days,** which summarizes the most important changes to make first.

Right after that, you'll see a closing section called **What You Can Expect**, which outlines the positive changes you should notice after implementing the plan for 4, 8, and 12 weeks.

Your Hormone Action Plan Worksheet

After reviewing the sample plans for inspiration, fill out the **Hormone Action Plan Worksheet** to build out your own plan. Scan to download this worksheet. Propose your plan to your healthcare team and ask for their input. Lead the conversation about your health, rather than taking a passive backseat.

Empowered and Ready for Action

Too many women stay stuck, not because they lack intelligence, desire, or effort but because they don't have a clear roadmap or because they're holding onto beliefs that don't serve them and that impede them from making the very changes they need to make. So many women feel anxious about their symptoms, unsure of the next steps, overwhelmed by conflicting advice, or simply resigned to the notion that "this must just be how it is." When women understand their hormonal landscape, everything changes. Their energy. Their presence. Their entire trajectory. And now you're standing in the doorway of that shift, ready to walk through.

My deepest hope is that this book has softened the fear, quieted the confusion, shifted your beliefs, and replaced overwhelm with a grounded, empowered sense of agency within you.

Your future self says "thank you" for the choices you are making today.

Conclusion

The whole time I was writing this book, two very important women remained at the top of my mind: my daughters, Madeleine and Emilia.

Although *Hormone Powered* is for every woman, I dedicated this book to my girls because they are my heart, my inspiration, and my motivation to be the best role model I can be.

When it comes to well-being, there is so much to say. So many nuances to address. So many personalized tweaks you can make. But if I could leave my girls, *and you*, the woman reading, with just five points to remember, this is what they would be.

Your Body Is Wise

Trust the signals your body is giving you—whether it's hunger or fullness, tiredness or vitality, pleasure or pain. Never let anyone tell you your symptoms are "all in your head" or that it's "normal" to feel unwell. It's not.

Symptoms are sacred messages from your body that bring important matters to your attention. When your body whispers, listen and act before it escalates into a shout.

Rest Is Not Laziness

Deep sleep. Slow mornings. Powering down your phone. Saying, "I'm honored to be invited, but I will need to decline," or "I'm fighting a cold and need to rest, so I won't be able to attend." These choices are the foundations of resilience, not weaknesses to apologize for.

When you take time to rest and recharge, you're not being apathetic, passive, or unambitious. You're powering up for the big work that's ahead of you.

With true rest comes true brilliance. Refueling more, rather than "pushing through," is the secret to unleashing your greatest work, whatever your work in this world may be, whether it's parenting, volunteering, running a medical practice, teaching, or anything else.

Exercising your ability to say "no" provides the ability to say "yes" to what your heart truly desires and the strength to throw your whole being into it.

Food Is Medicine and Joy

Nourish your hormones with real, vibrant food. Anchor your meals with protein, vegetables, nuts, seeds, healthy fats, and slow carbs. Choose whole, organic, and minimally processed options as often as you can. And savor that chocolate cake on your birthday, or that ice cream cone on the beach, and let this be medicine too.

Stress Is Not a Badge of Honor

Stress may seem honorable. We sometimes think feeling stressed out provides "proof" that we "care enough" to be worried, anxious, and dysregulated, that it's somehow "noble" to live in a state of constant tension. But chronic stress is not your friend. It doesn't fuel you. It only drains your power.

Learn what inspires you and calms you. Whether it's the circle of support you surround yourself with, music, breathwork, journaling, time in solitude, dancing, working out, or walking barefoot in the grass, find the best ways to settle your nervous system and release stress from your body.

Remember, too, that there are two forms of stress: distress, the unhealthy kind that wears you down, and eustress, the kind that challenges you in a positive way, that helps you grow and makes you stronger. Trust yourself to know the difference.

You Are Allowed to Change

Your cycles, your hormones, your dreams, goals, and priorities, all these things will shift.

Change doesn't mean something's wrong. It means you're evolving. Just as the moon transitions from the new moon to the full moon, you are meant to transform.

Your life will contain many seasons. Puberty, pregnancy, postpartum, perimenopause, menopause, and postmenopause are each challenging and beautiful in their own ways. Each phase is an opportunity to meet a new version of yourself and experience a new kind of power you have never known before.

If my daughters grow up knowing even a fraction of this, I'll know I've done my job as a mom. And if you, the woman reading, feel inspired to make even just *one* positive change based on what you've learned in *Hormone Powered*, then I will consider this book to be a success.

May you always live in tune with your heart, body, and purpose.

Wishing you a lifetime of radiant health.

—*Dr. Corina Dunlap*

Top 10 Concepts

Hormone Powered is a big, mighty, info-dense book. Want a quick list of the top 10 concepts to remember? Scan or visit http://drcorinadunlap.com/resources/ the code for your cheat sheet of the most essential points.

Resources

Scan or visit http://drcorinadunlap.com/resources/ to find free guides, worksheets, and other resources to support you. . .as you bring your hormones into balance and become your healthiest, most radiant self. You'll find:

The Hormone Type Assessment

- Do this online questionnaire to find out your primary Hormone Type: Caretaker, Achiever, or Survivor.
- Answer a series of questions about yourself. Get a personalized report with your results.

- Learn what your Hormone Type means about your beliefs and behavioral patterns, hormonal imbalances that are most likely for you, and the most powerful moves you can make to restore balance.

The Lab Testing Guide

Learn which lab tests are worth doing, where to get testing done, when to do them, and a few basic guidelines on how to interpret your results.

The Top 10 Concepts

A quick list of the top 10 concepts to remember from the book. This is your cheat sheet of the most essential points.

Bonus Chapter

A bonus chapter on the Hypothalamic-Pituitary-Thyroid-Adrenal-Ovarian Axis & Gut-Brain-Hormone Axis.

The Hormone Action Plan Worksheet

You read the book. Now create your plan! This worksheet includes sections you can fill in by hand, or type into, to create your personalized Hormone Action Plan.

Condition and Life-Stage Guides

Hoping to get pregnant? Seeking support in Perimenopause/Menopause? Trying to navigate PMOS, PMS/PMDD, Endometriosis, Postpartum, and more. These guides will provide a glimpse into how to use a holistic, naturopathic approach.

Work with Dr. Corina

If you struggle with…

Hormone concerns	Irregular periods or no period	Premenstrual syndrome (PMS) or premenstrual dysphoric disorder (PMDD)	Gastrointestinal health concerns
Unhealthy skin, nails, or hair	Polyendocrine metabolic ovarian syndrome (PMOS)	Subfertility/ Infertility	Perimenopause/ Menopause concerns
Thyroid concerns	Low libido	Painful sex	Vaginal dryness
Sleep concerns	Migraines	Anxiety, depression, or irritability	Weight fluctuation (gain or loss)
Acne	Joint pains	Osteopenia/ Osteoporosis	Adrenal concerns

Please visit www.NaturopathicByDesign.com to find out how you can work with Dr. Corina Dunlap or a provider from her team. You don't have to spend the rest of your life feeling unwell. Let us help.

You can also visit www.DrCorinaDunlap.com or email info@drcorinadunlap.com to inquire about booking Dr. Corina Dunlap for a speaking engagement or media appearance or to discuss another potential collaboration, such as engaging her services as a consultant or advisor for a healthcare product that your organization is launching. Reach out to explore possibilities.

A Small Request

Did this book make a positive difference in your life?

If so, please post a five-star review on Amazon, Goodreads, or wherever you prefer.

> "My favorite part of the book was. . ."

> "One thing that surprised me about this book was. . ."

> "This book inspired me to make some changes in my life, including. . ."

Why reviews are so important: the more reviews this book gets, the higher it rises in search results, which makes it easier for women to find it.

Millions of women suffer from conditions that arise due to hormonal imbalances. These are issues that could be solved, if they had the information and plan to do it.

Thank you for helping to bring this book into the hands of women who need it.

Acknowledgments

Hormone Powered would not exist without the village that helped to bring it to life.

I want to give immense thanks to. . .

- My husband, Amos, and my girls, Madeleine and Emilia, who were incredibly supportive throughout the research and writing process. You made the time away easier with your smiles, hugs, and encouragement. Knowing that you were rooting for me made the process so much more joyful.
- My publishing team at Wiley, including Sunnye Collins and Kim Wimpsett for thoughtful, eagle-eyed editing; Amy Fandrei for championing my vision; and Sophie Thompson for keeping everything organized and on track. Thank you for believing in me and the power of this book. I'm forever grateful that you helped me shepherd my first out into the world.
- My writing coach, Alexandra Franzen. From the first draft to the final version, you brought calm, encouraging energy and

helped me bring this project over the finish line. Writing a book while also running a busy women's health clinic, managing a team, serving patients, and raising kids is not easy, but you kept me on track with my deadlines. I honestly don't know how I could've done this without you.

- My team at Naturopathic by Design®. Getting to be your boss is one of the greatest privileges of my career. I'm blessed to work with such a stellar team of healthcare providers. We are helping women feel their absolute best at every stage of life, and I couldn't be more grateful!
- My mentors and colleagues in the healthcare field, Tori Hudson, Kimberly Windstar, and Heather Zwickey. For always believing in me and being the best role models.
- My dear friends and family who lent their homes for writing (in Hawaii, California, and Maine), playdates for my girls, and emotional support. You are the best!

To anyone I forgot to mention, know that you are appreciated deeply. Thank you.

About the Author

"I believe that health gives you resilience and strength. It allows you to live an inspired, abundant life. When you feel good, you can show up without restraint—as your most abundant shining self."

—*Dr. Corina Dunlap*

Dr. Corina Dunlap is a licensed naturopathic doctor, medical researcher, and expert in women's hormonal health. She is the founder of Naturopathic by Design®, a women's health clinic serving thousands of women in person and via telehealth nationwide.

What sets Dr. Dunlap apart is her ability to serve as a bridge between the best of conventional and natural medicine. Trained as both a clinician and a researcher, she combines the evidence-based rigor of modern research with the root-cause, whole-body thinking of naturopathic care. The result is a practice her patients describe as unlike anything they've experienced before, built on one simple mission: find the root cause, use the least invasive solution, and give women the tools they need to truly understand their bodies and feel their most radiant at every stage of life.

She earned her doctorate in naturopathic medicine and her master of science in integrative medicine research from the National University of Natural Medicine, where she later completed a postdoctoral women's health residency with rotations in gynecology, endocrinology, and reproductive health—followed by a postdoctoral research fellowship at the Helfgott Research Institute. Her research has been published in peer-reviewed medical journals, and she has served as a medical advisor and research consultant to LOLA, a leading women's wellness brand, and is co-owner of Beeya Wellness, an organic superfood company designed to support hormonal health.

She teaches reproductive medicine as an adjunct faculty member, speaks at national medical conferences, and has dedicated her career to a single belief: that when women truly understand their hormones, everything changes.

Dr. Dunlap lives in Maine, with her husband and two daughters. A former rock-climbing instructor and mountaineering guide, she traded her climbing gear for a stethoscope—but still believes the best medicine is found in nature. When she's not with patients or writing, you'll find her with a matcha in hand, lacing up her sneakers, and protecting her tech-free quiet time with family and loved ones.

Index